I0696181

The Ultimate Guide to Successful Weight Loss

Intentionally left blank

Table of Contents

Introduction..9

CHAPTER 1..10

Understanding the Basics of Weight Loss 10

    I. Introduction...11

        • The importance of understanding the basics of weight loss for successful weight management 11

        • Weight loss is a complex process that involves multiple factors................................11

    II. What is Weight Loss? 12

        • Definition of weight loss and how it works in the body....................................12

        • The concept of energy balance and how it relates to weight loss............................13

        • What is the role of metabolism in weight loss and how it can affect weight loss efforts 13

    III. Factors that Affect Weight Loss...14

        • Factors that can affect weight loss, including genetics, age, gender, and lifestyle habits......14

        • How these factors can impact weight loss efforts 15

    IV. Types of Weight Loss Programs 15

        • The different types of weight loss programs, including commercial programs, fad diets, and medically supervised programs...15

        • The pros and cons of each type of program 16

        • The importance of choosing a safe and effective weight loss program....................17

    V. Mindset and Weight Loss 18

        • The importance of mindset in weight loss 18

        • How mindset can affect motivation, behavior, and long-term success....................19

        • Strategies for developing a positive and sustainable mindset for weight loss 20

CHAPTER 2..21

Setting Realistic Goals 21

    I. Introduction...23

        • The importance of setting realistic goals for weight loss.....................................23

    II. Determining Realistic Goals..24

        • Tips for setting achievable weight loss goals 24

        • The importance of considering your current weight, lifestyle, and health................25

    III. Creating a Plan..26

- The role of planning in achieving weight loss goals 26
- Tips for creating a successful weight loss plan...27

IV. Staying Motivated 28
- Strategies for maintaining motivation throughout your weight loss journey.................28
- Celebrating successes and learning from setbacks 29

V. Tracking Progress 30
- The benefits of tracking progress towards weight loss goals 30
- Different methods for tracking progress 31

VI. Reassessing Goals...32
- The importance of periodically reassessing weight loss goals.............................32
- Making adjustments to your plan based on progress...33

CHAPTER 3 34

Creating a Healthy Diet Plan...34

I. Introduction..35

II. The Importance of a Healthy Diet Plan...35
- Health benefits of a healthy diet...35
- Factors that influence caloric intake 36
- Assessing your nutritional needs 36
- Creating a calorie deficit for weight loss..37

III. Choosing the Right Foods 38
- Food groups and the nutrients they provide 38
- Selecting nutrient-dense foods...38
- Reducing processed foods and sugars 39
- Incorporating a balance of macronutrients 40

IV. Building a Meal Plan...40
- Meal planning strategies...40
- Batch cooking and meal prep...41
- Planning meals that are convenient, affordable, and satisfying.............................42

V. Staying on Track 42
- Monitoring your progress 42
- Adjusting your plan as needed..43
- Seeking support from friends, family, or a healthcare professional 44

CHAPTER 4 45

Incorporating Exercise into Your Routine...45

    I. Introduction..47

        •   The importance of exercise in weight loss..47

        •   How exercise can improve overall health and well-being 47

    II. The Role of Exercise in Weight Loss and Weight Management 48

        •   Understanding the role of exercise in weight loss...................................48

        •   How exercise can help create a calorie deficit..49

        •   The benefits of regular exercise for weight management......................49

    III. Finding Your Ideal Exercise Routine 50

        •   The importance of finding an exercise routine that works for you 50

        •   Different types of exercise and their benefits 51

        •   How to choose an exercise program that fits your lifestyle and preferences 52

    IV. The Power of Consistency 53

        •   Incorporating exercise into your daily routine..53

        •   Tips for making exercise a regular habit 53

        •   The benefits of consistency in exercise...54

    V. Mastering Fitness 55

        •   Setting realistic goals for exercise...55

        •   The importance of tracking progress 56

        •   How to stay motivated and overcome obstacles....................................56

    VI. A Holistic Approach to Weight Loss 57

        •   Combining exercise with a healthy diet plan for maximum weight loss.............57

        •   How exercise and diet work together to achieve weight loss goals 58

        •   The benefits of a comprehensive weight loss plan 59

CHAPTER 5 61

Managing Stress and Getting Enough Sleep...61

    I. Introduction..62

        •   Importance of managing stress and getting enough sleep for overall well-being...........62

    II. Effects of Chronic Stress on Health 63

        •   Physical health problems associated with chronic stress 63

        •   Mental health problems associated with chronic stress..........................63

III. Importance of Sleep for Health 64

- Effects of chronic sleep deprivation on health 64

- Importance of sleep for brain function, memory consolidation, and physical restoration 65

IV. Strategies for Managing Stress and Improving Sleep..65

- Stress-reducing activities such as meditation and deep breathing exercises 65

- Establishing a regular sleep schedule and creating a sleep-conducive environment 66

CHAPTER 6 67

Staying Motivated and Overcoming Obstacles 67

I. Introduction..68

- The importance of staying motivated to achieve fitness goals...68

- Overcoming obstacles that may arise during the journey to better health and fitness 68

II. Key Strategies for Achieving Realistic Fitness Goals..69

- Setting realistic goals and expectations for yourself 69

- Breaking down larger goals into smaller, more manageable steps 70

- Focusing on progress rather than perfection...70

III. Strategies for making exercise a regular and enjoyable part of your lifestyle 71

- Finding an exercise routine that you enjoy and look forward to...71

- Varying your workouts to prevent boredom and maintain interest..71

- Incorporating exercise into your daily routine..72

IV. Strategies for Staying Motivated and Overcoming Obstacles in Your Fitness Journey................72

- Staying accountable by tracking progress and celebrating successes 72

- Seeking support from friends, family, or a professional coach..73

- Overcoming common obstacles, such as lack of time, motivation, or energy.........................73

V. Key Components of a Sustainable Fitness Routine..74

- Recognizing the importance of rest and recovery in preventing burnout...............................74

- Incorporating mindfulness practices, such as meditation or deep breathing, into your routine to   reduce stress and increase focus...74

- Adjusting your approach as needed, and being willing to try new things to keep yourself engaged and motivated...74

CHAPTER 7 76

Maintaining Weight Loss and Preventing Relapse 76

I. Introduction..78

- Importance of weight loss maintenance..78
- Challenges of weight loss maintenance 78

II. Creating a Supportive Environment 79
- Surrounding yourself with positive influences..79
- Finding a support system 79
- Staying accountable 79

III. Sticking to Healthy Habits..80
- Consistency in exercise routine 80
- Making healthy food choices 80
- Balancing calorie intake and expenditure..80
- Staying hydrated 81

IV. Addressing Emotional Eating...81
- Identifying triggers..81
- Finding alternative coping mechanisms..81
- Seeking professional help when needed 81

V. Coping with Setbacks and Challenges 82
- Recognizing and learning from mistakes 82
- Dealing with plateaus...82
- Overcoming weight loss plateaus 83
- Dealing with negative self-talk 84

VI. Keeping the Motivation and Momentum Going 85
- Setting new goals 85
- Rewarding yourself for accomplishments..85
- Celebrating progress 86

References:..88

Intentionally left blank

Introduction

Welcome to The Ultimate Guide to Successful Weight Loss.

This book is designed to help you achieve your weight loss goals in a healthy, sustainable way. You will learn everything you need to know about losing weight, from creating a healthy diet and exercise plan, to managing stress and getting enough sleep.

Welcome to The Ultimate Guide to Successful Weight Loss. Losing weight can be a challenging and sometimes frustrating journey, but it doesn't have to be. With the right information and strategies, you can achieve your weight loss goals in a healthy, sustainable way. This book is designed to provide you with everything you need to know to create a personalized weight loss plan that works for you.

We will cover the basic principles of weight loss, including how calories work, the role of macronutrients, and the importance of exercise. You'll learn how to set realistic goals and create a personalized plan that takes into account your current weight, lifestyle, and personal preferences. We'll provide tips for creating a healthy eating plan, including which foods to include and avoid, and how to handle social situations that involve food. You'll also learn about the different types of exercise that can help you lose weight and improve your overall health, as well as strategies for staying motivated and overcoming obstacles.

But weight loss isn't just about diet and exercise. Stress and lack of sleep can also have a negative impact on weight loss, so we'll cover strategies for managing stress and getting enough sleep. And once you've achieved your weight loss goals, the challenge becomes maintaining your new weight and preventing relapse. We'll provide practical tips for maintaining your weight loss over the long-term, as well as strategies for dealing with setbacks and preventing relapse.

Whether you're just starting your weight loss journey or you've been struggling for a while, The Ultimate Guide to Successful Weight Loss has everything you need to succeed. So, let's get started!

CHAPTER 1

Understanding the Basics of Weight Loss

I. Introduction

- The importance of understanding the basics of weight loss for successful weight management
- Weight loss is a complex process that involves multiple factors

II. What is Weight Loss?

- Definition of weight loss and how it works in the body
- The concept of energy balance and how it relates to weight loss
- What is the role of metabolism in weight loss and how it can affect weight loss efforts

III. Factors that Affect Weight Loss

- Factors that can affect weight loss, including genetics, age, gender, and lifestyle habits
- How these factors can impact weight loss efforts

V. Types of Weight Loss Programs

- The different types of weight loss programs, including commercial programs, fad diets, and medically supervised programs
- The pros and cons of each type of program
- The importance of choosing a safe and effective weight loss program

VI. Mindset and Weight Loss

- The importance of mindset in weight loss
- How mindset can affect motivation, behavior, and long-term success
- Strategies for developing a positive and sustainable mindset for weight loss

I. Introduction

- **The importance of understanding the basics of weight loss for successful weight management**

Understanding the basics of weight loss is crucial for successful weight management because it provides a solid foundation of knowledge and skills needed to make sustainable changes to one's lifestyle habits. When someone has a clear understanding of how weight loss works and the factors that affect it, they are better equipped to make informed decisions about their diet and exercise habits.

For example, knowing the importance of calories and energy balance can help someone make smarter food choices and control their portion sizes. Understanding the role of metabolism in weight loss can help someone identify any underlying issues that may be hindering their progress, such as a slow metabolism or hormonal imbalances. Knowing the impact of lifestyle factors such as stress and sleep on weight loss can also help someone make adjustments to their daily routine to support their weight loss goals.

Furthermore, understanding the basics of weight loss can help someone navigate the overwhelming amount of information and misinformation that exists around weight loss. With so many fad diets and weight loss programs available, it can be difficult to know what advice to follow. However, when someone has a solid understanding of the basics of weight loss, they can better evaluate the validity of different weight loss approaches and choose ones that are safe and effective.

In short, understanding the basics of weight loss is essential for successful weight management because it empowers someone with the knowledge and skills needed to make sustainable lifestyle changes that support their weight loss goals.

- **Weight loss is a complex process that involves multiple factors**

There are several factors that can impact weight loss efforts, including genetics, age, gender, and lifestyle habits. Here are some ways in which these factors can affect weight loss efforts:

1. Genetics: Genetics can influence body composition, metabolism, and other factors that can impact weight loss. Some people may have a genetic predisposition to store more fat or have a slower metabolism, which can make weight loss more difficult.
2. Age: As we age, our metabolism slows down, and we tend to lose muscle mass. This can make it harder to lose weight and easier to gain weight. Additionally, hormonal changes that occur with age can also impact weight loss efforts.
3. Gender: Men and women have different body compositions, hormonal profiles, and metabolic rates, which can impact weight loss efforts. For example, men tend to have more muscle mass than women, which can make it easier for them to lose weight.

4. Lifestyle habits: Lifestyle habits such as diet, exercise, sleep, and stress management can all impact weight loss efforts. Eating a diet high in processed foods and sugar, for example, can make it harder to lose weight, while regular exercise can help to burn calories and build muscle.

It's important to note that while these factors can impact weight loss efforts, they are not determinative. With the right mindset, knowledge, and habits, it is possible to successfully lose weight regardless of these factors. By focusing on creating a healthy and sustainable lifestyle that supports weight loss, individuals can overcome any challenges posed by genetics, age, gender, or lifestyle habits.

II. What is Weight Loss?

- **Definition of weight loss and how it works in the body**

Weight loss refers to the reduction in body weight, which can occur due to a decrease in body fat, muscle mass, or body fluid. The most common form of weight loss is fat loss, which is achieved by creating a calorie deficit through a combination of diet and exercise.

In order to understand how weight loss works in the body, it's important to understand the concept of energy balance. Energy balance refers to the relationship between the calories consumed through food and the calories burned through physical activity and metabolic processes.

When someone consumes more calories than their body needs to maintain its current weight, the excess calories are stored as fat. Conversely, when someone consumes fewer calories than their body needs, the body must use stored fat as energy to make up for the deficit. This leads to weight loss.

In order to lose one pound of body fat, it is necessary to create a calorie deficit of approximately 3,500 calories. This can be achieved through a combination of reducing calorie intake through diet and increasing calorie expenditure through exercise. For example, if someone reduces their calorie intake by 500 calories per day and burns an additional 500 calories per day through exercise, they can create a daily calorie deficit of 1,000 calories, which can lead to a weight loss of two pounds per week.

It's important to note that weight loss is not just about reducing calories. The quality of the calories consumed also plays a role in weight loss. Consuming a diet high in nutrient-dense whole foods such as fruits, vegetables, lean proteins, and healthy fats can help support weight loss and overall health. In addition, regular exercise can help to burn calories, build muscle, and improve overall health and fitness.

- **The concept of energy balance and how it relates to weight loss**

Energy balance is a concept that refers to the relationship between the number of calories consumed through food and the number of calories burned through physical activity and metabolic processes. When energy intake (calories consumed) equals energy expenditure (calories burned), a person is said to be in energy balance and will maintain their current weight.

When someone consumes more calories than their body needs for energy, the excess calories are stored as fat. Over time, this can lead to weight gain. Conversely, when someone consumes fewer calories than their body needs for energy, the body must use stored fat for energy, which can lead to weight loss.

The key to successful weight loss is creating a calorie deficit, which means consuming fewer calories than the body needs to maintain its current weight. This can be achieved by reducing calorie intake through a healthy diet and increasing calorie expenditure through exercise.

It's important to note that the quality of calories consumed is also important for weight loss and overall health. Consuming a diet high in nutrient-dense whole foods such as fruits, vegetables, lean proteins, and healthy fats can help support weight loss and overall health. In addition, regular exercise can help to burn calories, build muscle, and improve overall health and fitness.

Overall, the concept of energy balance is crucial to understanding weight loss. By creating a calorie deficit through a combination of diet and exercise, it is possible to lose weight and improve overall health and wellbeing.

- **What is the role of metabolism in weight loss and how it can affect weight loss efforts**

Metabolism refers to the chemical processes that occur in the body to maintain life. It involves the conversion of food into energy that can be used by the body for various functions, including physical activity, digestion, and circulation.

The rate at which the body burns calories to produce energy is known as the metabolic rate. The metabolic rate can be influenced by a number of factors, including genetics, age, body composition, and activity level.

A person's metabolism can affect their weight loss efforts in a number of ways. For example, someone with a slower metabolic rate may burn fewer calories at rest and during physical activity, making it more difficult for them to create a calorie deficit and lose weight. This can be compounded by factors such as age, which can naturally lead to a slower metabolic rate.

However, there are ways to boost metabolism and support weight loss efforts. One effective way is through regular exercise, which can help to build muscle mass and increase the metabolic rate. Consuming a diet high in protein can also support metabolism, as the body requires more energy to digest and metabolize protein than it does for carbohydrates or fats.

It's important to note that while metabolism can play a role in weight loss, it's not the only factor. Creating a calorie deficit through a combination of diet and exercise is still the most effective way to achieve weight loss. However, understanding the role of metabolism can help individuals tailor their approach to weight loss and optimize their results.

III. Factors that Affect Weight Loss

- **Factors that can affect weight loss, including genetics, age, gender, and lifestyle habits**

Weight loss is a complex process that can be influenced by a variety of factors. Some of the key factors that can affect weight loss include genetics, age, gender, and lifestyle habits.

1. Genetics: Your genetic makeup plays a significant role in determining your body weight and body composition. Studies have shown that genes can affect your metabolism, appetite, and how your body stores and uses fat. Some people may have a genetic predisposition to obesity, making it more difficult for them to lose weight.
2. Age: As you age, your body's metabolism slows down, which can make it more difficult to lose weight. This is because your body burns fewer calories at rest, so you need to consume fewer calories or increase physical activity to maintain the same weight. Additionally, muscle mass tends to decrease as you age, which can further slow down your metabolism.
3. Gender: Men and women have different body compositions, with men generally having more muscle mass and higher levels of testosterone, which can help with weight loss. However, women tend to have a higher percentage of body fat, which can make weight loss more challenging.
4. Lifestyle habits: Lifestyle habits such as diet and physical activity are critical factors in weight loss. Consuming a diet high in calories, saturated fats, and added sugars can contribute to weight gain, while eating a diet rich in fruits, vegetables, lean protein, and whole grains can support weight loss. Physical activity is also essential, as it helps to burn calories, build muscle, and improve overall health.

Other factors that can affect weight loss include medical conditions, medications, and sleep patterns. It is important to speak with a healthcare provider before starting any weight loss program to identify any underlying health conditions that may need to be addressed. Additionally, working with a registered dietitian or certified personal trainer can help you develop a personalized weight loss plan that takes into account your unique needs and challenges.

- **How these factors can impact weight loss efforts**

1. Genetics: Genetics can affect weight loss efforts by influencing how your body responds to different diets and physical activity levels. For example, some people may have a genetic predisposition to store fat more easily, making it more difficult to lose weight. Additionally, genetics can affect appetite and metabolism, which can impact how many calories your body burns and how hungry you feel.
2. Age: Age can impact weight loss efforts because as you get older, your body's metabolism slows down, meaning you burn fewer calories at rest. This can make it more difficult to create a calorie deficit, which is necessary for weight loss. Additionally, as you age, you may experience a decrease in muscle mass, which can further decrease your metabolism.
3. Gender: Gender can impact weight loss efforts because men and women have different body compositions, which can affect how many calories they burn and how much muscle they have. Men tend to have higher muscle mass and a higher metabolic rate, making it easier for them to lose weight. Women, on the other hand, tend to have a higher percentage of body fat and a lower metabolic rate, making weight loss more challenging.
4. Lifestyle habits: Lifestyle habits such as diet and physical activity are critical to weight loss efforts. Eating a healthy, balanced diet and engaging in regular physical activity can help create a calorie deficit and support weight loss. Conversely, consuming a diet high in calories and engaging in little physical activity can make it difficult to lose weight and may even lead to weight gain.

Overall, these factors can impact weight loss efforts by influencing metabolism, appetite, and body composition. Understanding these factors and how they affect weight loss can help individuals develop personalized weight loss plans that are effective and sustainable.

IV. Types of Weight Loss Programs

- **The different types of weight loss programs, including commercial programs, fad diets, and medically supervised programs**

There are several types of weight loss programs, each with its own approach and level of support. Some of the most common types of weight loss programs include commercial programs, fad diets, and medically supervised programs.

1. Commercial programs: Commercial weight loss programs are often designed to be easy to follow, with pre-packaged meals, supplements, and support from coaches or peers. These programs may include Weight Watchers, Jenny Craig, or Nutrisystem. Commercial programs typically require payment, and the cost can vary depending on the program.

2. Fad diets: Fad diets are often trendy and promise quick weight loss results, but they are not always sustainable or healthy. These diets may eliminate certain food groups or require strict calorie restrictions, such as the ketogenic diet or the grapefruit diet. While some people may see short-term weight loss success with fad diets, they are not a sustainable or healthy approach to weight loss.
3. Medically supervised programs: Medically supervised weight loss programs are designed and supervised by healthcare professionals, such as doctors or registered dietitians. These programs may include personalized meal plans, medication, and behavioral therapy. Medically supervised programs are typically more expensive than commercial programs or fad diets, but they may provide a more comprehensive and personalized approach to weight loss.

When choosing a weight loss program, it's important to consider your individual needs and goals. A program that works well for one person may not be the best fit for another. It's also important to choose a program that promotes sustainable, healthy habits rather than quick fixes or drastic measures. Before starting any weight loss program, it's a good idea to consult with a healthcare provider to ensure it is safe and appropriate for you.

- **The pros and cons of each type of program**

Here are some pros and cons of each type of weight loss program:

1. Commercial programs:

Pros:

- Pre-packaged meals and snacks can be convenient and save time.
- Support from coaches and peers can provide motivation and accountability.
- Programs are often structured and easy to follow.

Cons:

- Programs can be expensive.
- Meals and snacks may be highly processed and may not provide a balanced, nutritious diet.
- Some programs may not provide enough support for long-term weight loss success.

2. Fad diets:

Pros:

- Some people may see quick weight loss results.
- Many fad diets are free or low-cost.

- Some diets, such as the Mediterranean diet, may promote healthy eating habits.

Cons:

- Fad diets are often not sustainable or healthy in the long term.
- Many diets eliminate entire food groups, which can lead to nutrient deficiencies.
- Some diets may be difficult to follow, leading to feelings of deprivation and frustration.

3. Medically supervised programs:

Pros:

- Programs are designed and supervised by healthcare professionals, which can provide a personalized and comprehensive approach to weight loss.
- Programs may provide medication and behavioral therapy to support long-term weight loss success.
- Programs may provide support for addressing underlying medical conditions that can contribute to weight gain.

Cons:

- Programs can be expensive.
- Some programs may require frequent appointments and interventions, which may be time-consuming.
- Programs may not provide the same level of convenience as commercial programs.

Overall, the most effective weight loss program is one that is sustainable, healthy, and tailored to your individual needs and preferences. It's important to consider the pros and cons of each type of program and choose one that fits your lifestyle and goals. Consulting with a healthcare provider can also help you determine the best approach for your individual needs.

- **The importance of choosing a safe and effective weight loss program**

Choosing a safe and effective weight loss program is important for several reasons:

1. Health risks: Some weight loss programs may be unsafe or even dangerous, especially if they require extreme calorie restriction, elimination of entire food groups, or the use of untested supplements. These approaches can lead to nutrient deficiencies, electrolyte imbalances, and other health risks.
2. Sustainability: Sustainable weight loss is more likely to occur when you adopt healthy habits that you can maintain in the long term. Programs that promote quick weight loss

through drastic measures are often not sustainable, and weight regain may occur once you stop following the program.

3. Psychological well-being: Weight loss programs can impact your mental health, and programs that promote extreme calorie restriction or eliminate entire food groups can lead to feelings of deprivation and frustration. It's important to choose a program that promotes a balanced, healthy approach to weight loss to support your psychological well-being.
4. Financial considerations: Some weight loss programs can be expensive, and it's important to consider the financial implications of a program before starting. Choosing a safe and effective weight loss program that fits within your budget can reduce stress and support long-term success.

When choosing a weight loss program, it's important to research the program thoroughly and consider the credentials of the individuals or organizations promoting the program. Consulting with a healthcare provider can also help you determine whether a program is safe and appropriate for your individual needs. Ultimately, the best weight loss program is one that supports sustainable, healthy habits that can be maintained in the long term.

V. Mindset and Weight Loss

- **The importance of mindset in weight loss**

Mindset plays a crucial role in weight loss because it shapes our thoughts, beliefs, and behaviors around food and physical activity. Developing a healthy and positive mindset towards weight loss can help you stay motivated, overcome obstacles, and achieve long-term success. Here are some ways in which mindset can impact weight loss:

1. Motivation: When you have a positive mindset, you are more likely to stay motivated to lose weight. Instead of focusing on what you can't eat, focus on the positive changes you are making for your health and well-being.
2. Self-Efficacy: A positive mindset can help you build self-efficacy, or the belief in your ability to achieve your weight loss goals. When you have confidence in yourself, you are more likely to stick to your healthy habits and persevere through challenges.
3. Resilience: Weight loss is not always a linear process, and setbacks can happen. A positive mindset can help you bounce back from setbacks and stay focused on your goals.
4. Stress Management: Stress can often trigger unhealthy eating habits, such as emotional eating. A positive mindset can help you manage stress in a healthier way, such as through exercise, meditation, or other relaxation techniques.
5. Sustainable Habits: Mindset is important for developing sustainable habits that can support long-term weight loss. Instead of focusing on short-term diets or fads, a positive mindset can help you make gradual, healthy changes to your lifestyle that you can maintain over time.

In summary, developing a positive mindset is crucial for weight loss success. By focusing on healthy habits, building self-efficacy, and managing stress, you can develop a sustainable approach to weight loss that supports your overall health and well-being.

- **How mindset can affect motivation, behavior, and long-term success**

Mindset can have a significant impact on motivation, behavior, and long-term success in weight loss. Here's how:

1. Motivation: Your mindset can influence your motivation to lose weight. A positive mindset can help you stay motivated by focusing on the positive aspects of weight loss, such as improved health and self-confidence. On the other hand, a negative mindset can lead to feelings of frustration and hopelessness, making it more difficult to stay motivated.
2. Behavior: Mindset can also affect your behaviors related to weight loss. A positive mindset can help you adopt healthy habits, such as eating a balanced diet and engaging in regular exercise. Conversely, a negative mindset can lead to unhealthy behaviors, such as emotional eating and a sedentary lifestyle.
3. Long-term success: Mindset is crucial for achieving long-term success in weight loss. A positive mindset can help you overcome obstacles and setbacks, stay committed to your goals, and make sustainable lifestyle changes. In contrast, a negative mindset can lead to giving up on your weight loss journey altogether or resorting to unhealthy and unsustainable methods for weight loss.

Here are some specific ways in which mindset can impact long-term success in weight loss:

- Perseverance: A positive mindset can help you persevere through challenges and setbacks, such as a weight loss plateau or a slip-up in your diet or exercise routine.
- Self-efficacy: A positive mindset can help you build self-efficacy, or the belief in your ability to achieve your weight loss goals. This can lead to greater confidence in your ability to make healthy choices and maintain a healthy lifestyle.
- Mindful eating: Mindset can also affect how you approach food. A positive mindset can help you develop a more mindful approach to eating, such as paying attention to hunger and fullness cues, rather than relying on emotional triggers.
- Sustainable habits: Mindset is crucial for developing sustainable habits that can support long-term weight loss. A positive mindset can help you adopt healthy habits that you can maintain over time, rather than resorting to short-term diets or fads.

In summary, mindset can significantly impact motivation, behavior, and long-term success in weight loss. By cultivating a positive mindset and focusing on sustainable habits, you can increase your chances of achieving your weight loss goals and maintaining a healthy lifestyle.

- **Strategies for developing a positive and sustainable mindset for weight loss**

Developing a positive and sustainable mindset is essential for weight loss success. Here are some strategies that can help you cultivate a positive and sustainable mindset for weight loss:

1. Focus on the positives: Instead of focusing on what you can't eat or the challenges you may face, focus on the positive changes you are making for your health and well-being. Celebrate your successes, no matter how small they may seem, and recognize that every healthy choice you make is a step in the right direction.
2. Set realistic goals: Setting realistic and achievable goals can help you build confidence in your ability to succeed. Be specific about what you want to achieve and break down your goals into smaller, more manageable steps.
3. Practice self-compassion: Be kind and compassionate to yourself, especially when you face setbacks or challenges. Instead of being self-critical or judgmental, practice self-compassion by treating yourself with the same kindness and understanding you would offer to a friend.
4. Practice mindfulness: Mindfulness can help you develop a more positive and sustainable mindset by increasing your awareness of your thoughts, emotions, and behaviors. Practice mindfulness techniques, such as meditation or deep breathing, to help you stay focused on the present moment and reduce stress.
5. Build a support network: Surround yourself with people who support and encourage your weight loss goals. Join a support group, work with a coach or trainer, or enlist the help of family and friends who share your commitment to healthy living.
6. Focus on sustainable habits: Rather than focusing on short-term diets or fads, focus on building sustainable habits that you can maintain over time. Make gradual changes to your lifestyle, such as increasing your physical activity, eating a balanced diet, and getting enough sleep, that support your overall health and well-being.

In summary, developing a positive and sustainable mindset is essential for weight loss success. By focusing on the positives, setting realistic goals, practicing self-compassion, practicing mindfulness, building a support network, and focusing on sustainable habits, you can cultivate a

positive and sustainable mindset that supports your weight loss goals and overall health and well-being.

CHAPTER 2

Setting Realistic Goals

I. Introduction

- The importance of setting realistic goals for weight loss

II. Determining Realistic Goals

- Tips for setting achievable weight loss goals

- The importance of considering your current weight, lifestyle, and health

III. Creating a Plan

- The role of planning in achieving weight loss goals

- Tips for creating a successful weight loss plan

IV. Staying Motivated

- Strategies for maintaining motivation throughout your weight loss journey

- Celebrating successes and learning from setbacks

V. Tracking Progress

- The benefits of tracking progress towards weight loss goals

- Different methods for tracking progress

VI. Reassessing Goals

- The importance of periodically reassessing weight loss goals

- Making adjustments to your plan based on progress

I. Introduction

Losing weight can be a challenging and overwhelming journey, and setting realistic goals is a crucial aspect of achieving success. It can be tempting to set lofty goals and expect instant results, but the truth is that sustainable weight loss takes time and effort. In this chapter, we will explore the importance of setting realistic goals for weight loss and provide practical tips and strategies to help you achieve them. Whether you're starting your weight loss journey or looking to make progress towards your existing goals, this chapter will guide you in establishing achievable milestones and developing a plan to reach them. By setting realistic goals and creating a roadmap for success, you can build the foundation for a healthier and happier life.

- **The importance of setting realistic goals for weight loss**

Setting realistic goals is an essential aspect of achieving success in weight loss. Here are some reasons why:

1. Avoiding frustration and disappointment

When you set unattainable weight loss goals, you may feel frustrated and defeated when you don't see immediate progress. This can lead to giving up on your weight loss journey altogether. However, if you set realistic goals that are achievable within a reasonable timeframe, you'll feel more motivated to continue working towards them.

2. Increasing the likelihood of success

Setting realistic weight loss goals increases the likelihood of success. If you set goals that are too challenging or unrealistic, you're less likely to achieve them, which can be demotivating. However, when you set achievable goals, you'll have a greater chance of success, and each accomplishment will motivate you to keep going.

3. Improving overall health

Losing weight can reduce the risk of chronic conditions such as heart disease, diabetes, and high blood pressure. By setting realistic weight loss goals and working towards them, you'll be taking an important step towards a healthier and happier life.

4. Building confidence

Setting and achieving realistic weight loss goals can also boost your confidence and self-esteem. When you achieve your goals, you'll feel proud of yourself, which can translate to other areas of your life. This positive mindset can help you tackle other challenges and improve your overall wellbeing.

By setting realistic weight loss goals, you'll avoid frustration and disappointment, increase the likelihood of success, improve your overall health, and build confidence. In the next section, we'll discuss some tips for setting achievable weight loss goals.

II. Determining Realistic Goals

- **Tips for setting achievable weight loss goals**

When it comes to setting weight loss goals, it's important to be realistic and specific. Here are some tips to help you set achievable weight loss goals:

1. Set a realistic timeframe

It's essential to set a realistic timeframe for your weight loss goals. Losing weight too quickly can be unhealthy and unsustainable, and it's essential to have patience and persistence. Set a timeframe that allows you to make progress while maintaining a healthy and balanced lifestyle.

2. Set specific goals

Setting specific weight loss goals can help you track progress and stay motivated. Instead of setting a broad goal such as "lose weight," break it down into smaller, specific goals such as "lose 1-2 pounds per week" or "reduce my waist circumference by 2 inches."

3. Make your goals measurable

Making your weight loss goals measurable can help you track progress and adjust your approach if needed. Consider tracking your progress through regular weigh-ins or measurements of body fat percentage or waist circumference.

4. Consider non-scale goals

While weight loss is an important aspect of overall health, consider setting non-scale goals such as improving your fitness level or increasing the number of servings of fruits and vegetables you consume daily. These goals can help you focus on healthy behaviors that will contribute to weight loss and overall wellbeing.

5. Celebrate accomplishments

Finally, it's important to celebrate your accomplishments along the way. Recognize the hard work and effort that goes into achieving your weight loss goals, no matter how small they may seem. Celebrating accomplishments can help keep you motivated and committed to achieving your goals.

By setting a realistic timeframe, specific and measurable goals, considering non-scale goals, and celebrating accomplishments, you can set achievable weight loss goals and make progress towards a healthier and happier life.

- **The importance of considering your current weight, lifestyle, and health**

When setting weight loss goals, it's crucial to consider your current weight, lifestyle, and health. Here are some reasons why:

1. Safety

Your current weight, lifestyle, and health can impact the safety of your weight loss journey. Rapid weight loss or extreme diets can be dangerous, especially for those with underlying health conditions. Before starting any weight loss program, it's essential to consult with a healthcare provider to ensure it's safe and appropriate for you.

2. Realistic expectations

Considering your current weight, lifestyle, and health can help you set realistic expectations for your weight loss journey. If you're significantly overweight, it may take longer to achieve your goals than someone who only needs to lose a few pounds. Additionally, if you have a sedentary lifestyle or underlying health conditions, you may need to start with small changes and gradually increase your activity level and intensity.

3. Motivation

Setting weight loss goals that are appropriate for your current weight, lifestyle, and health can help keep you motivated. If you set unrealistic goals, you may become discouraged when progress is slow or non-existent. However, setting achievable goals that align with your current abilities and lifestyle can help you see progress and stay motivated to continue working towards your goals.

4. Sustainable lifestyle changes

Finally, considering your current weight, lifestyle, and health can help you make sustainable lifestyle changes. Weight loss is not just about shedding pounds; it's about adopting healthy habits that you can maintain long-term. By considering your current abilities and lifestyle, you can make changes that are realistic and sustainable, leading to lasting results.

By considering your current weight, lifestyle, and health, you can set safe, realistic, and motivating weight loss goals that lead to sustainable lifestyle changes and lasting results. In the next section, we'll discuss some common pitfalls to avoid when setting weight loss goals.

III. Creating a Plan

- **The role of planning in achieving weight loss goals**

Planning plays a crucial role in achieving weight loss goals. Here are some reasons why:

1. Establishing a roadmap

Planning helps establish a roadmap for achieving your weight loss goals. By breaking down your goals into smaller, manageable steps, you can create a plan that outlines what you need to do to achieve them. A plan helps you stay on track and gives you a sense of direction, making it easier to stay motivated and focused on your goals.

2. Anticipating obstacles

When you have a plan in place, you can anticipate obstacles and plan for how to overcome them. For example, if you know you tend to snack when you're stressed, you can plan ahead and have healthy snacks on hand to avoid reaching for junk food. Anticipating obstacles and planning for them can help you stay on track and avoid setbacks.

3. Accountability

A plan helps hold you accountable for your actions. When you have a clear plan in place, you know what you need to do to achieve your goals. This can make it easier to stay accountable to yourself and to others, such as a friend or support group.

4. Tracking progress

A plan can also help you track your progress. By setting specific goals and breaking them down into smaller steps, you can track your progress and see how far you've come. This can be motivating and help you stay focused on your goals.

5. Making adjustments

Finally, a plan allows you to make adjustments as needed. As you track your progress, you may find that some strategies work better than others. By having a plan in place, you can make adjustments to your approach and continue working towards your goals.

By creating a plan that outlines specific goals, anticipates obstacles, holds you accountable, tracks progress, and allows for adjustments, you can set yourself up for success in achieving your weight loss goals. In the next section, we'll discuss common pitfalls to avoid when setting weight loss goals.

- **Tips for creating a successful weight loss plan**

Creating a successful weight loss plan requires careful consideration and planning. Here are some tips to help you create a plan that works for you:

1. Set specific, measurable, and achievable goals

To create a successful weight loss plan, you need to set specific, measurable, and achievable goals. For example, instead of setting a vague goal to "lose weight," set a specific goal to "lose 10 pounds in 3 months." This gives you a clear target to work towards and helps you track your progress.

2. Make gradual changes

Making too many changes too quickly can be overwhelming and unsustainable. Instead, make gradual changes to your diet and exercise routine. For example, start by adding more fruits and vegetables to your diet or taking a 15-minute walk each day. Gradually increase the intensity and duration of your exercise over time.

3. Find a support system

Having a support system can make a significant difference in achieving your weight loss goals. This could be a friend or family member who also wants to lose weight, a support group, or a healthcare professional. Having someone to talk to, share your progress with, and hold you accountable can make it easier to stay on track.

4. Plan for obstacles

Anticipating obstacles and planning for how to overcome them is essential for success. For example, if you know you'll be attending a social event with unhealthy food, plan ahead by eating a healthy meal beforehand or bringing a healthy snack with you. Having a plan in place can help you stay on track and avoid setbacks.

5. Celebrate successes

Celebrating your successes, no matter how small, can help you stay motivated and focused on your goals. For example, if you've reached a milestone, treat yourself to a non-food reward, such as a new workout outfit or a massage.

By setting specific, measurable, and achievable goals, making gradual changes, finding a support system, planning for obstacles, and celebrating successes, you can create a successful weight loss plan that works for you. In the next section, we'll discuss some common pitfalls to avoid when setting weight loss goals.

IV. Staying Motivated

- **Strategies for maintaining motivation throughout your weight loss journey**

Maintaining motivation is critical to achieving your weight loss goals. Here are some strategies that can help you stay motivated:

1. Keep track of your progress

Tracking your progress can be an effective way to stay motivated. This could include weighing yourself regularly, taking measurements of your body, or keeping a food and exercise diary. Seeing progress, no matter how small, can help you stay focused and motivated.

2. Focus on non-scale victories

While it's important to have a weight loss goal, it's also essential to focus on non-scale victories. These are achievements that are not related to the number on the scale, such as being able to run a mile without stopping, fitting into a smaller size of clothing, or feeling more energized. Focusing on these achievements can help you stay motivated even if your weight loss progress slows down.

3. Surround yourself with positivity

Negativity can be a significant demotivator. Surrounding yourself with positivity can help you stay motivated and focused on your goals. This could include following social media accounts that promote a healthy lifestyle, listening to uplifting music, or spending time with supportive friends and family members.

4. Reward yourself

Rewarding yourself can be a great way to stay motivated. Choose rewards that are not food-related, such as treating yourself to a spa day, going to a movie, or buying a new outfit. Rewards can be a powerful motivator, but make sure they align with your weight loss goals and are not counterproductive.

5. Be kind to yourself

Weight loss is a journey, and setbacks are inevitable. Being kind to yourself, forgiving yourself for mistakes, and treating yourself with compassion can help you stay motivated and avoid giving up. Remember that progress, not perfection, is the goal.

By keeping track of your progress, focusing on non-scale victories, surrounding yourself with positivity, rewarding yourself, and being kind to yourself, you can maintain motivation throughout your weight loss journey. In the next section, we'll discuss some common obstacles that can derail your weight loss progress and how to overcome them.

- **Celebrating successes and learning from setbacks**

Weight loss is a journey with ups and downs, and it's important to celebrate successes and learn from setbacks along the way. Here are some tips on how to do this:

1. Celebrate your successes

When you achieve a weight loss goal, no matter how small, take the time to celebrate it. This could mean treating yourself to a non-food reward or sharing your success with supportive friends and family members. Celebrating your successes can help you stay motivated and feel proud of your progress.

2. Learn from your setbacks

Setbacks are inevitable on the weight loss journey, but they don't have to derail your progress. Instead of beating yourself up for a setback, take the time to reflect on what happened and what you can learn from it. Did you experience a stressful event that caused you to overeat? Did you skip a workout because you were feeling tired or unmotivated? By understanding what led to the setback, you can create a plan to avoid it in the future.

3. Use setbacks as motivation

Instead of letting setbacks discourage you, use them as motivation to keep going. Think of setbacks as temporary obstacles on your journey towards your weight loss goals. Use them as an opportunity to reflect on your progress, adjust your plan if necessary, and come back stronger.

4. Focus on the bigger picture

Remember that weight loss is not just about the number on the scale. It's about improving your health, feeling more confident, and living a happier life. When setbacks happen, focus on the bigger picture and remember why you started your weight loss journey in the first place.

By celebrating your successes, learning from your setbacks, using setbacks as motivation, and focusing on the bigger picture, you can navigate the ups and downs of the weight loss journey with resilience and determination. In the final section, we'll summarize the key points of the chapter and provide some additional resources for achieving your weight loss goals.

V. Tracking Progress

- **The benefits of tracking progress towards weight loss goals**

Tracking your progress towards your weight loss goals can provide several benefits, including:

1. Motivation

When you track your progress, you can see how far you've come and feel motivated to keep going. Seeing progress can be a powerful motivator, especially during times when you may feel discouraged or unmotivated.

2. Accountability

Tracking your progress can help keep you accountable to your goals. When you have a record of your progress, you can see where you may need to adjust your plan to stay on track.

3. Identifying patterns and trends

Tracking your progress can help you identify patterns and trends in your weight loss journey. For example, you may notice that you tend to overeat when you're stressed or that you consistently have trouble sticking to your exercise routine on certain days of the week. By identifying these patterns, you can create strategies to overcome them and improve your chances of success.

4. Celebrating successes

Tracking your progress can also help you celebrate your successes along the way. By recording your progress, you can see how far you've come and celebrate each milestone achieved.

There are several ways to track progress, including measuring your weight, taking measurements of your body, and keeping a food and exercise diary. Choose a method that works best for you and make it a regular part of your weight loss journey.

By tracking your progress towards your weight loss goals, you can stay motivated, accountable, and identify patterns and trends that can help you adjust your plan for success. In the final section, we'll summarize the key points of the chapter and provide some additional resources for achieving your weight loss goals.

- **Different methods for tracking progress**

There are several methods for tracking progress towards your weight loss goals. The best method for you will depend on your personal preferences and what works best for you. Here are some common methods for tracking progress:

1. Measuring your weight

Weighing yourself regularly is a common way to track progress towards your weight loss goals. You can use a scale at home or weigh yourself at a gym or health clinic. It's important to keep in mind that your weight can fluctuate throughout the day and from day to day, so it's best to weigh yourself at the same time and under the same conditions each time.

2. Taking measurements of your body

Another way to track progress is by taking measurements of your body. This can include measuring your waist, hips, arms, and thighs. Measuring your body can give you a better understanding of how your body is changing even if the scale doesn't show a significant change.

3. Keeping a food and exercise diary

Keeping a food and exercise diary is a helpful way to track your progress towards your weight loss goals. By recording what you eat and how much you exercise, you can identify areas where you may need to make adjustments to your plan. You can also look back at your diary to see how far you've come and celebrate your successes.

4. Using a fitness tracker

Fitness trackers are electronic devices that track your physical activity, including steps taken, distance traveled, and calories burned. Some fitness trackers also monitor your heart rate and sleep patterns. Using a fitness tracker can help you stay motivated and accountable to your exercise goals.

Choose a method or combination of methods that works best for you and make it a regular part of your weight loss journey. By tracking your progress towards your weight loss goals, you can stay motivated and accountable, identify patterns and trends, and celebrate your successes along the way. In the final section, we'll summarize the key points of the chapter and provide some additional resources for achieving your weight loss goals.

VI. Reassessing Goals

- **The importance of periodically reassessing weight loss goals**

While setting realistic goals and creating a solid plan is important, it's also essential to periodically reassess your weight loss goals to make sure they are still achievable and realistic. This is because your body and circumstances may change over time, and what was once a reasonable goal may no longer be realistic or safe.

Here are some reasons why it's important to periodically reassess your weight loss goals:

1. Changes in health

If you have a health condition, such as high blood pressure, diabetes, or heart disease, you may need to adjust your weight loss goals to ensure they align with your doctor's recommendations. Similarly, if you experience a health setback, such as an injury or illness, you may need to reassess your goals to ensure they are still attainable.

2. Changes in lifestyle

Your lifestyle can also affect your weight loss goals. For example, if you start a new job that requires more sedentary activity, you may need to adjust your exercise goals to accommodate for the decrease in physical activity. Similarly, if you experience a major life event, such as a pregnancy or a move to a new city, you may need to reassess your goals to ensure they are still feasible given your new circumstances.

3. Changes in progress

As you make progress towards your weight loss goals, it's important to reassess them periodically to ensure they are still challenging but achievable. If you find yourself consistently meeting or exceeding your goals, it may be time to set new, more challenging goals. On the other hand, if you're consistently falling short of your goals, it may be time to adjust them to ensure they are realistic and achievable.

By periodically reassessing your weight loss goals, you can ensure they remain realistic, achievable, and aligned with your health, lifestyle, and progress. This can help you stay motivated and on track towards achieving your ultimate weight loss goals.

- **Making adjustments to your plan based on progress**

As you work towards your weight loss goals, it's important to monitor your progress regularly and make adjustments to your plan as needed. This can help you stay motivated and on track towards achieving your ultimate weight loss goals.

Here are some tips for making adjustments to your weight loss plan based on your progress:

1. Monitor your progress

Regularly tracking your progress can help you identify areas where you're making progress and areas where you may need to make adjustments to your plan. Some common ways to track progress include weighing yourself regularly, taking measurements of your body, and keeping a food and exercise journal.

2. Celebrate your successes

When you reach a milestone or make progress towards your weight loss goals, take the time to celebrate your successes. This can help you stay motivated and remind you of the progress you've made.

3. Learn from setbacks

Setbacks are a natural part of any weight loss journey. Instead of getting discouraged, use setbacks as an opportunity to learn and adjust your plan. Ask yourself what went wrong and what you can do differently in the future to avoid similar setbacks.

4. Make adjustments to your plan

Based on your progress and what you've learned from setbacks, make adjustments to your weight loss plan as needed. This may involve adjusting your goals, changing your exercise routine, or modifying your diet.

5. Stay motivated

Finally, it's important to stay motivated throughout your weight loss journey. Surround yourself with supportive friends and family, reward yourself for making progress, and remind yourself of the benefits of achieving your weight loss goals.

By monitoring your progress, celebrating your successes, learning from setbacks, making adjustments to your plan, and staying motivated, you can achieve your weight loss goals and improve your overall health and well-being.

CHAPTER 3

Creating a Healthy Diet Plan

I. Introduction

II. The Importance of a Healthy Diet Plan

- Health benefits of a healthy diet
- Factors that influence caloric intake
- Assessing your nutritional needs
- Creating a calorie deficit for weight loss

III. Choosing the Right Foods

- Food groups and the nutrients they provide
- Selecting nutrient-dense foods
- Reducing processed foods and sugars
- Incorporating a balance of macronutrients

IV. Building a Meal Plan

- Meal planning strategies
- Batch cooking and meal prep
- Planning meals that are convenient, affordable, and satisfying

V. Staying on Track

- Monitoring your progress
- Adjusting your plan as needed
- Seeking support from friends, family, or a healthcare professional

I. Introduction

Maintaining a healthy weight is crucial for overall health and wellbeing, but with the abundance of conflicting information and fad diets out there, creating a sustainable and effective diet plan can be overwhelming. A healthy diet is key to successful weight loss, but understanding the principles of a healthy diet and developing a plan that works for you can be a challenge.

This chapter will guide you through the process of creating a healthy diet plan that supports your weight loss goals and improves your overall health and wellbeing. We will explore the critical components of a healthy diet plan, including the importance of a healthy diet, assessing your nutritional needs, choosing the right foods, building a meal plan, and staying on track.

By the end of this chapter, you will have the knowledge and tools you need to create a sustainable and enjoyable diet plan that supports your weight loss goals and improves your overall health and wellbeing. Let's begin by understanding the importance of a healthy diet plan for successful weight loss.

II. The Importance of a Healthy Diet Plan

- **Health benefits of a healthy diet**

A healthy diet provides numerous health benefits beyond just weight loss. Here are some examples of the health benefits of a healthy diet:

1. Reduced risk of chronic diseases: A diet that is rich in fruits, vegetables, whole grains, lean proteins, and healthy fats can reduce the risk of chronic diseases such as heart disease, stroke, type 2 diabetes, and some forms of cancer.
2. Improved gut health: A healthy diet that includes plenty of fiber can improve gut health by promoting healthy digestion, reducing inflammation, and supporting the growth of healthy gut bacteria.
3. Increased energy levels: Consuming a balanced diet can provide the body with the necessary nutrients to support energy production, leading to increased energy levels and improved physical performance.
4. Improved cognitive function: A healthy diet can improve cognitive function by providing the brain with the necessary nutrients to support memory, concentration, and overall brain health.
5. Stronger immune system: A diet that is rich in vitamins, minerals, and other nutrients can strengthen the immune system, reducing the risk of infections and illnesses.
6. Better sleep: A balanced diet can promote better sleep by improving sleep quality and reducing the risk of sleep disorders such as insomnia.

Overall, a healthy diet can provide numerous health benefits beyond just weight loss, including reduced risk of chronic diseases, improved gut health, increased energy levels, improved cognitive function, a stronger immune system, and better sleep.

- **Factors that influence caloric intake**

Caloric intake is influenced by various factors, including:

1. Basal metabolic rate (BMR): BMR refers to the number of calories your body burns at rest to maintain basic bodily functions such as breathing, circulation, and temperature regulation. BMR is influenced by factors such as age, gender, body size, and body composition, and it can vary from person to person.
2. Physical activity: The amount of physical activity you engage in can significantly affect your caloric intake. Higher levels of physical activity require more calories to fuel the body, while sedentary lifestyles require fewer calories.
3. Diet composition: The types of foods you consume can influence caloric intake. Foods that are high in fat and sugar are typically more calorie-dense than foods that are high in fiber and protein.
4. Environmental factors: The environment you are in can also affect your caloric intake. For example, the availability and accessibility of food can influence how much you consume. Social factors such as eating with friends and family can also influence how much you eat.
5. Psychological factors: Psychological factors such as stress, emotions, and habits can also affect caloric intake. Emotional eating, for example, can lead to consuming more calories than your body needs.
6. Medications and medical conditions: Certain medications and medical conditions can also affect caloric intake. For example, some medications can increase appetite, while others can suppress it. Medical conditions such as thyroid disorders can also affect metabolism and caloric intake.

Overall, caloric intake is influenced by various factors, and understanding these factors can help individuals develop a healthy diet plan that supports their weight loss goals and overall health and wellbeing.

- **Assessing your nutritional needs**

Assessing your nutritional needs is an important step in creating a healthy diet plan for weight loss. It involves evaluating your current diet and determining which nutrients you may be deficient in or consuming in excess. Here are some ways to assess your nutritional needs:

1. Calculate your calorie needs: Determining your daily calorie needs is the first step in creating a healthy diet plan. You can use online calculators or consult with a registered

dietitian to determine your daily calorie needs based on your age, gender, height, weight, and activity level.

2. Evaluate your current diet: Keeping a food diary can help you evaluate your current diet and identify areas where you may need to make changes. Look for patterns in your diet, such as consuming too much saturated fat or not enough fiber, and make adjustments accordingly.

3. Identify nutrient deficiencies: Certain nutrient deficiencies can lead to health problems, so it is important to identify any deficiencies in your diet. A registered dietitian can help you evaluate your diet and identify any nutrient deficiencies.

4. Consider your health status: Certain health conditions may require specific dietary modifications. For example, individuals with high blood pressure may need to reduce their sodium intake, while those with celiac disease may need to avoid gluten.

5. Consult with a registered dietitian: A registered dietitian can provide personalized nutrition advice based on your individual needs and goals. They can help you evaluate your diet, identify areas where you may need to make changes, and provide guidance on creating a healthy diet plan for weight loss.

Overall, assessing your nutritional needs is an important step in creating a healthy diet plan for weight loss. By evaluating your current diet, identifying nutrient deficiencies, and considering your health status, you can create a personalized diet plan that supports your weight loss goals and overall health and wellbeing.

- **Creating a calorie deficit for weight loss**

Creating a calorie deficit is a key factor in weight loss. It means that you are burning more calories than you are consuming, which forces your body to use stored fat as energy. Here are some ways to create a calorie deficit for weight loss:

1. Reduce calorie intake: Reducing your calorie intake is the most effective way to create a calorie deficit. You can do this by making changes to your diet, such as reducing portion sizes, choosing lower calorie foods, and limiting high-calorie snacks and drinks.

2. Increase physical activity: Increasing physical activity can help you burn more calories and create a calorie deficit. You can do this by incorporating more exercise into your daily routine, such as going for a walk or jog, joining a fitness class, or participating in a team sport.

3. Combine diet and exercise: Combining a healthy diet with regular exercise is the most effective way to create a calorie deficit and achieve weight loss. Aim to consume a healthy, balanced diet that is rich in nutrients and low in calories, while also incorporating regular exercise into your routine.

4. Monitor progress: Monitoring your progress is important to ensure that you are creating a calorie deficit and achieving weight loss. Keep track of your calorie intake

and physical activity using a food diary or fitness tracker, and adjust your diet and exercise routine as needed to continue making progress.

It's important to note that creating a calorie deficit for weight loss should be done in a healthy and sustainable way. Severe calorie restriction or excessive exercise can be harmful to your health and may not lead to long-term weight loss. Consulting with a healthcare provider or registered dietitian can help you create a safe and effective calorie deficit plan that supports your weight loss goals and overall health and wellbeing.

III. Choosing the Right Foods

- **Food groups and the nutrients they provide**

There are five main food groups, each of which provides different nutrients that are essential for good health. Here's a breakdown of each food group and the nutrients they provide:

1. Fruits: Fruits are a good source of vitamins, minerals, and fiber. They are rich in vitamin C, potassium, and folate. Fruits are also a good source of antioxidants, which help protect your body against cell damage.
2. Vegetables: Vegetables are packed with vitamins, minerals, and fiber. They are a good source of vitamin A, vitamin C, potassium, and folate. Vegetables also contain phytochemicals, which are plant compounds that have health benefits.
3. Grains: Grains are a good source of carbohydrates, which provide energy for your body. Whole grains are also a good source of fiber, which helps promote digestive health. Grains are rich in B vitamins, such as thiamin, niacin, and riboflavin.
4. Protein foods: Protein foods are important for building and repairing tissues in your body. They are a good source of essential amino acids, which are the building blocks of protein. Protein foods include meat, poultry, fish, beans, peas, nuts, and seeds.
5. Dairy: Dairy products are a good source of calcium, which is important for strong bones and teeth. Dairy products also provide vitamin D, which helps your body absorb calcium. Low-fat or fat-free dairy products are also a good source of protein.

It's important to consume a variety of foods from each food group to ensure that you get all of the nutrients your body needs. A balanced diet that includes a variety of fruits, vegetables, grains, protein foods, and dairy can help promote good health and reduce the risk of chronic diseases.

- **Selecting nutrient-dense foods**

Selecting nutrient-dense foods is an important part of creating a healthy diet plan. Nutrient-dense foods are foods that provide a high amount of nutrients relative to their calorie content. These foods are rich in vitamins, minerals, fiber, and other essential nutrients that your body needs to function properly. Here are some tips for selecting nutrient-dense foods:

1. Choose whole, minimally processed foods: Whole foods, such as fruits, vegetables, whole grains, lean protein sources, and low-fat dairy, are more nutrient-denser than processed foods. Processed foods are often high in calories, unhealthy fats, sugar, and sodium, but low in nutrients.
2. Read food labels: Reading food labels can help you identify nutrient-dense foods. Look for foods that are low in saturated fat, trans fat, and added sugars, and high in fiber, vitamins, and minerals.
3. Focus on variety: Eating a variety of nutrient-dense foods can help ensure that you get all of the essential nutrients your body needs. Aim to include a variety of fruits, vegetables, whole grains, lean proteins, and low-fat dairy in your diet.
4. Be mindful of portion sizes: Even nutrient-dense foods can contribute to weight gain if consumed in large quantities. Be mindful of portion sizes and try to balance your calorie intake with your physical activity levels.
5. Consider nutrient supplements: In some cases, it may be difficult to get all of the essential nutrients you need from food alone. Consider taking a daily multivitamin or other nutrient supplement to help fill any nutrient gaps in your diet.

By selecting nutrient-dense foods, you can ensure that your body gets the essential nutrients it needs to function properly, while also supporting your overall health and wellbeing.

- **Reducing processed foods and sugars**

Reducing processed foods and sugars is an important aspect of creating a healthy diet plan. Processed foods are often high in unhealthy fats, sodium, and added sugars, while providing few essential nutrients. Similarly, consuming too much sugar can contribute to weight gain, increase the risk of chronic diseases like diabetes, and negatively impact overall health. Here are some tips for reducing processed foods and sugars in your diet:

1. Choose whole foods: Whole foods, such as fruits, vegetables, whole grains, lean proteins, and low-fat dairy, are naturally low in added sugars and unhealthy fats. By focusing on whole foods, you can reduce your intake of processed foods.
2. Read food labels: Reading food labels can help you identify the amount of added sugars and unhealthy fats in processed foods. Look for foods that are low in added sugars and unhealthy fats, and high in fiber, vitamins, and minerals.
3. Limit sugary beverages: Sugary beverages, such as soda, juice, and sports drinks, can be a major source of added sugars in your diet. Opt for water, unsweetened tea, or other low-sugar beverages instead.
4. Use natural sweeteners: If you want to add sweetness to your food or drinks, consider using natural sweeteners like honey, maple syrup, or stevia, which are lower in calories and have a lower glycemic index than table sugar.
5. Cook at home: Cooking at home allows you to control the ingredients and cooking methods used in your meals. By preparing your own meals, you can reduce your intake of processed foods and sugars.

By reducing processed foods and sugars in your diet, you can improve your overall health and reduce the risk of chronic diseases. Aim to focus on whole foods, read food labels, limit sugary beverages, use natural sweeteners, and cook at home to create a healthier diet plan.

- **Incorporating a balance of macronutrients**

Incorporating a balance of macronutrients is important for creating a healthy diet plan. Macronutrients are the nutrients that your body needs in large amounts to function properly, including carbohydrates, proteins, and fats. Each macronutrient serves a specific purpose in the body, and incorporating a balance of all three can help support overall health and wellbeing. Here are some tips for incorporating a balance of macronutrients in your diet:

1. Carbohydrates: Carbohydrates provide your body with energy and are an important source of fiber. Aim to include complex carbohydrates, such as whole grains, fruits, and vegetables, in your diet.
2. Proteins: Proteins are important for building and repairing tissues, as well as for maintaining a healthy immune system. Aim to include lean protein sources, such as poultry, fish, beans, and nuts, in your diet.
3. Fats: Fats are important for brain function and hormone production, as well as for providing energy. Aim to include healthy fats, such as those found in nuts, seeds, avocado, and fatty fish, in your diet.
4. Balance your portions: Aim to balance your portions of carbohydrates, proteins, and fats at each meal. For example, a balanced meal might include a serving of lean protein, a serving of complex carbohydrates, and a serving of healthy fats.
5. Avoid fad diets: Fad diets that severely restrict or eliminate one or more macronutrients can be harmful to your health. Instead, focus on creating a balanced and varied diet that incorporates all three macronutrients.

By incorporating a balance of macronutrients in your diet, you can support your overall health and wellbeing. Aim to include complex carbohydrates, lean protein sources, and healthy fats in your meals, and balance your portions of each macronutrient. Avoid fad diets that eliminate or severely restrict one or more macronutrients, and focus on creating a balanced and sustainable diet plan.

IV. Building a Meal Plan

- **Meal planning strategies**

Meal planning strategies can be helpful for creating a healthy diet plan that is both balanced and sustainable. Here are some tips for meal planning:

1. Set aside time for planning: Set aside time each week to plan your meals for the upcoming week. This can help you stay organized and ensure that you have all the ingredients you need on hand.
2. Choose a variety of foods: Aim to include a variety of foods in your meal plan, including fruits, vegetables, whole grains, lean proteins, and healthy fats. This can help ensure that you are getting all the nutrients your body needs.
3. Consider your schedule: When planning your meals, consider your schedule and choose recipes that are quick and easy to prepare on busy days.
4. Batch cook: Batch cooking can save you time and ensure that you have healthy meals ready to go throughout the week. Consider preparing large batches of meals that you can portion out for the week ahead.
5. Shop with a list: Create a shopping list based on your meal plan and stick to it when grocery shopping. This can help you avoid impulse buys and ensure that you have all the ingredients you need on hand.
6. Use leftovers: Leftovers can be a great way to save time and reduce food waste. Consider incorporating leftovers into your meal plan for the week.

By implementing these meal planning strategies, you can create a healthy and sustainable diet plan. Remember to choose a variety of foods, consider your schedule, batch cook, shop with a list, and use leftovers. With a little planning and preparation, you can enjoy healthy and delicious meals throughout the week.

- **Batch cooking and meal prep**

Batch cooking and meal prep are meal planning strategies that involve preparing meals in advance to save time and ensure that you have healthy meals on hand throughout the week.

Batch cooking involves preparing large batches of meals or ingredients, such as roasted vegetables or cooked grains, that can be stored in the fridge or freezer and used in meals throughout the week. For example, you might prepare a large batch of chili or soup that can be portioned out for lunches or dinners throughout the week. Batch cooking can save time and reduce the need for daily meal prep.

Meal prep involves preparing individual meals or components of meals in advance. This might involve cooking chicken breasts, roasting vegetables, and portioning out servings of grains or salads into individual containers for easy grab-and-go meals throughout the week. Meal prep can be helpful for those with busy schedules who want to ensure that they have healthy meals on hand without having to spend time cooking each day.

Both batch cooking and meal prep can be helpful strategies for creating a healthy diet plan that is sustainable and easy to maintain. By preparing meals in advance, you can save time, reduce food waste, and ensure that you have healthy and delicious meals on hand throughout the week.

- **Planning meals that are convenient, affordable, and satisfying**

When planning a healthy diet, it's important to consider factors beyond just nutrition. Meals that are convenient, affordable, and satisfying are more likely to be sustainable in the long term. Here are some tips for planning meals that meet these criteria:

1. Choose recipes that are quick and easy to prepare: Look for recipes that can be made in 30 minutes or less, or that can be prepared in advance and reheated later.
2. Use ingredients that are affordable: Look for ingredients that are in season and on sale to help keep costs down. Frozen fruits and vegetables can also be a budget-friendly option.
3. Opt for filling foods: Choose foods that are high in fiber and protein, as these can help you feel fuller for longer. Examples include whole grains, beans, lentils, nuts, and seeds.
4. Include variety: Don't be afraid to mix things up and try new recipes and ingredients. This can help keep meals interesting and satisfying.
5. Plan for leftovers: Leftovers can be a great way to save time and money. When planning meals, consider making extra servings that can be eaten for lunch the next day or frozen for later.
6. Keep snacks on hand: Having healthy snacks on hand can help prevent overeating and reduce the need for convenience foods. Examples include fresh fruit, cut-up vegetables, hummus, and yogurt.

By planning meals that are convenient, affordable, and satisfying, you can create a healthy diet plan that is both enjoyable and sustainable. Remember to choose quick and easy recipes, use affordable ingredients, opt for filling foods, include variety, plan for leftovers, and keep healthy snacks on hand.

V. Staying on Track

- **Monitoring your progress**

Monitoring your progress is an important aspect of creating a healthy diet plan. By tracking your progress, you can determine if you are on track to meet your goals, identify areas where you may need to make adjustments, and celebrate your successes.

Here are some tips for monitoring your progress:

1. Keep a food diary: Writing down what you eat can help you become more aware of your eating habits and identify areas where you may need to make changes. You can use a paper diary, a mobile app, or a website to track your food intake.

2. Weigh yourself regularly: Regular weigh-ins can help you track your progress and identify if you need to make changes to your diet or exercise routine. However, it's important to keep in mind that weight can fluctuate for various reasons, so it's important to look at trends over time rather than focusing on day-to-day changes.
3. Take measurements: In addition to weighing yourself, taking measurements such as waist circumference and body fat percentage can provide a more complete picture of your progress.
4. Track your exercise: Keeping track of your physical activity can help you ensure that you are getting enough exercise to support your weight loss goals. You can use a fitness tracker, a mobile app, or a website to track your exercise.
5. Celebrate your successes: Celebrating your successes, no matter how small, can help keep you motivated and on track. For example, you might reward yourself with a new workout outfit or a massage for reaching a certain milestone.

By monitoring your progress, you can ensure that you are on track to meet your goals and make adjustments as needed. Remember to keep a food diary, weigh yourself regularly, take measurements, track your exercise, and celebrate your successes.

- **Adjusting your plan as needed**

Adjusting your plan as needed is an important part of creating a successful and sustainable healthy diet plan. As you progress through your weight loss journey, you may encounter challenges or changes in your lifestyle that require you to make adjustments to your plan. Here are some tips for adjusting your plan as needed:

1. Be flexible: It's important to be flexible and open to making changes as needed. Recognize that your needs and circumstances may change over time, and be willing to adjust your plan accordingly.
2. Evaluate your progress regularly: Regularly assessing your progress can help you identify areas where you may need to make changes. Keep track of your weight, measurements, and other markers of progress, and use this information to evaluate your plan and make adjustments as needed.
3. Seek support: If you're struggling to make progress or are unsure how to adjust your plan, seek support from a healthcare professional, registered dietitian, or weight loss support group. They can provide guidance and support to help you stay on track.
4. Experiment with new foods and recipes: Adding variety to your diet can help keep you motivated and prevent boredom. Experiment with new foods and recipes to keep things interesting and enjoyable.
5. Don't give up: Remember that setbacks and challenges are a normal part of the weight loss journey. Don't give up if you experience a setback or struggle to make progress. Instead, focus on making small, sustainable changes to your plan and celebrating your successes along the way.

By being flexible, regularly evaluating your progress, seeking support, experimenting with new foods and recipes, and staying committed to your goals, you can adjust your plan as needed and create a healthy diet plan that works for you.

- **Seeking support from friends, family, or a healthcare professional**

Seeking support from friends, family, or a healthcare professional can be a valuable tool in creating a successful and sustainable healthy diet plan. Here are some ways that different types of support can help:

1. Friends and family: Having a support system of friends and family can help you stay motivated and accountable. They can offer encouragement, help you stay on track, and provide emotional support when you're feeling discouraged.
2. Registered dietitian: A registered dietitian can provide expert guidance on creating a healthy diet plan that meets your individual needs and preferences. They can help you develop a personalized meal plan, provide education on nutrition and healthy eating, and offer ongoing support and accountability.
3. Weight loss support group: Joining a weight loss support group can provide a sense of community and support from others who are also on a weight loss journey. These groups can provide motivation, accountability, and tips and strategies for success.
4. Healthcare professional: If you have underlying health conditions or are taking medication that affects your weight, it's important to consult with a healthcare professional before starting a weight loss plan. They can help you determine safe and effective goals, provide guidance on nutrition and exercise, and monitor your progress to ensure you're staying healthy and safe.

Incorporating support from friends, family, or a healthcare professional can be an important part of creating a healthy diet plan that works for you. By seeking support and guidance, you can increase your chances of success and make sustainable changes for a healthier lifestyle.

CHAPTER 4

Incorporating Exercise into Your Routine

I. Introduction

- The importance of exercise in weight loss
- How exercise can improve overall health and well-being

II. The Role of Exercise in Weight Loss and Weight Management

- Understanding the role of exercise in weight loss
- How exercise can help create a calorie deficit
- The benefits of regular exercise for weight management

III. Finding Your Ideal Exercise Routine

- The importance of finding an exercise routine that works for you
- Different types of exercise and their benefits
- How to choose an exercise program that fits your lifestyle and preferences

IV. The Power of Consistency

- Incorporating exercise into your daily routine
- Tips for making exercise a regular habit
- The benefits of consistency in exercise

V. Mastering Fitness

- Setting realistic goals for exercise
- The importance of tracking progress
- How to stay motivated and overcome obstacles

VI. A Holistic Approach to Weight Loss

- Combining exercise with a healthy diet plan for maximum weight loss

- How exercise and diet work together to achieve weight loss goals
- The benefits of a comprehensive weight loss plan

I. Introduction

- **The importance of exercise in weight loss**

Exercise is a critical component of weight loss for several reasons. Here are some of the key ways in which exercise can help with weight loss:

1. Burns calories: Exercise helps to burn calories, which can help to create a calorie deficit that leads to weight loss. When you exercise, your body uses energy (calories) to fuel the activity. The more intense the activity, the more calories you'll burn.
2. Increases metabolism: Regular exercise can help to boost your metabolism, which is the rate at which your body burns calories. This means that even when you're not exercising, your body will be burning more calories than it would if you were sedentary.
3. Preserves muscle: When you lose weight, you not only lose fat, but you may also lose muscle. Regular exercise can help to preserve muscle mass, which is important for maintaining a healthy metabolism.
4. Improves insulin sensitivity: Exercise can help to improve your body's sensitivity to insulin, which is a hormone that regulates blood sugar levels. When your body is more sensitive to insulin, it can better regulate blood sugar levels, which can help to prevent weight gain and promote weight loss.
5. Reduces stress: Exercise can help to reduce stress levels, which can be beneficial for weight loss. Stress can cause your body to release cortisol, a hormone that can promote weight gain, particularly in the abdominal area.
6. Boosts mood: Exercise has been shown to boost mood and reduce symptoms of depression and anxiety. This can be important for weight loss, as people who are in a good mood are more likely to make healthy choices.

Overall, exercise is an important component of weight loss. By burning calories, boosting metabolism, preserving muscle mass, improving insulin sensitivity, reducing stress, and boosting mood, exercise can help to promote sustainable weight loss and improve overall health.

- **How exercise can improve overall health and well-being**

Exercise can provide numerous benefits for overall health and well-being. Here are some of the ways in which exercise can improve health:

1. Reduces the risk of chronic diseases: Regular exercise can help to reduce the risk of chronic diseases such as heart disease, diabetes, and some forms of cancer. Exercise

can improve cardiovascular health, lower blood pressure, reduce inflammation, and improve insulin sensitivity.

2. Helps to manage weight: Exercise can help to create a calorie deficit, which can lead to weight loss. Even moderate exercise can be effective in helping to manage weight, particularly when combined with a healthy diet.

3. Improves cardiovascular health: Exercise can help to improve cardiovascular health by strengthening the heart and improving circulation. This can help to reduce the risk of heart disease, stroke, and other cardiovascular problems.

4. Increases muscle strength and endurance: Exercise can help to increase muscle strength and endurance, which can make everyday activities easier and reduce the risk of injury.

5. Improves bone health: Exercise can help to improve bone density, which is important for preventing osteoporosis and reducing the risk of fractures.

6. Improves mental health: Exercise has been shown to improve mood, reduce symptoms of depression and anxiety, and reduce stress levels. This can be particularly beneficial for overall well-being.

7. Improves cognitive function: Exercise has been shown to improve cognitive function and reduce the risk of cognitive decline with aging.

Overall, exercise can have a significant impact on overall health and well-being. By reducing the risk of chronic diseases, helping to manage weight, improving cardiovascular health, increasing muscle strength and endurance, improving bone health, and improving mental and cognitive health, exercise can help to promote a longer, healthier, and more fulfilling life.

II. The Role of Exercise in Weight Loss and Weight Management

- **Understanding the role of exercise in weight loss**

Exercise plays an essential role in weight loss by burning calories and increasing metabolism. When you exercise, your body burns calories to fuel the activity. The more intense the activity, the more calories you burn. This calorie burning can create a calorie deficit, which is necessary for weight loss.

In addition to burning calories, exercise can also increase metabolism. This is the rate at which your body burns calories. Regular exercise can help to boost your metabolism, which means that even when you're not exercising, your body will be burning more calories than it would if you were sedentary. This increased metabolism can help to support weight loss efforts.

Furthermore, exercise can help to preserve muscle mass, which is essential for maintaining a healthy metabolism. When you lose weight, you not only lose fat, but you may also lose muscle. Regular exercise can help to preserve muscle mass, which can help to keep your metabolism high and promote long-term weight loss.

It's worth noting that exercise alone may not be enough to achieve significant weight loss. A healthy diet is also crucial for weight loss, as calorie intake plays a critical role in creating a calorie deficit. However, exercise can be a powerful tool in conjunction with a healthy diet for achieving and maintaining weight loss.

Overall, exercise is a crucial component of weight loss, as it can help to burn calories, increase metabolism, and preserve muscle mass. By incorporating regular exercise into a weight loss plan, individuals can achieve sustainable weight loss and promote overall health and well-being.

- **How exercise can help create a calorie deficit**

Exercise can help to create a calorie deficit, which is necessary for weight loss. A calorie deficit occurs when you burn more calories than you consume. This creates an energy imbalance that forces your body to use stored fat as fuel, resulting in weight loss.

Exercise can help to create a calorie deficit in several ways:

1. Burns calories: Exercise burns calories, which can help to create a calorie deficit. The more intense the exercise, the more calories you burn.
2. Increases metabolism: Exercise can help to boost metabolism, which is the rate at which your body burns calories. Regular exercise can help to increase metabolism, even when you're not exercising. This means that your body will be burning more calories throughout the day, helping to create a calorie deficit.
3. Helps to build muscle: Muscle burns more calories than fat, even when you're not exercising. Exercise can help to build muscle, which can increase your resting metabolic rate, helping to burn more calories throughout the day.
4. Reduces appetite: Exercise can help to reduce appetite, particularly for high-calorie, high-fat foods. This can help to reduce calorie intake, which can contribute to a calorie deficit.
5. Increases energy expenditure: Exercise can increase energy expenditure, which is the amount of energy your body uses to perform daily activities. By increasing energy expenditure, exercise can help to create a calorie deficit.

Overall, exercise can be a powerful tool for creating a calorie deficit, which is essential for weight loss. By burning calories, boosting metabolism, building muscle, reducing appetite, and increasing energy expenditure, exercise can help to create an energy imbalance that promotes sustainable weight loss.

- **The benefits of regular exercise for weight management**

Regular exercise can be beneficial for weight management in many ways. Here are some of the benefits of regular exercise for weight management:

1. Burns calories: Exercise burns calories, which can help to create a calorie deficit and support weight loss. The more intense the exercise, the more calories you burn.
2. Increases metabolism: Exercise can help to increase metabolism, which is the rate at which your body burns calories. Regular exercise can help to increase metabolism, even when you're not exercising. This means that your body will be burning more calories throughout the day, helping to support weight management efforts.
3. Helps to preserve muscle mass: Exercise can help to preserve muscle mass, which is important for maintaining a healthy metabolism. When you lose weight, you not only lose fat but may also lose muscle. Regular exercise can help to preserve muscle mass, which can help to keep your metabolism high and promote long-term weight management.
4. Reduces body fat: Exercise can help to reduce body fat, particularly visceral fat, which is the type of fat that accumulates around your organs and is associated with an increased risk of chronic diseases.
5. Improves insulin sensitivity: Exercise can help to improve insulin sensitivity, which is important for managing blood sugar levels and reducing the risk of diabetes.
6. Reduces stress: Exercise can help to reduce stress levels, which can be beneficial for weight management. Stress can trigger overeating or poor food choices, and regular exercise can help to combat stress and reduce the likelihood of these behaviors.
7. Improves overall health: Regular exercise can help to improve overall health, reducing the risk of chronic diseases such as heart disease, diabetes, and some forms of cancer. Improved health can also support weight management efforts.

Overall, regular exercise can be highly beneficial for weight management. By burning calories, increasing metabolism, preserving muscle mass, reducing body fat, improving insulin sensitivity, reducing stress, and improving overall health, exercise can help to support sustainable weight management efforts.

III. Finding Your Ideal Exercise Routine

- **The importance of finding an exercise routine that works for you**

Finding an exercise routine that works for you is essential for creating a sustainable and enjoyable exercise habit. Here are some reasons why:

1. Consistency: When you find an exercise routine that you enjoy and that fits into your schedule, you're more likely to stick with it. Consistency is key to achieving and maintaining the benefits of exercise, including weight management, improved health, and overall well-being.
2. Enjoyment: When you enjoy your exercise routine, you're more likely to look forward to it and feel motivated to do it. This can help to make exercise a positive part of your life rather than a chore or burden.

3. Individual needs: Everyone has different fitness levels, preferences, and physical needs. Finding an exercise routine that works for you can help you to meet your individual needs and avoid injury or burnout.
4. Variety: Finding an exercise routine that works for you doesn't mean doing the same thing every day. Incorporating a variety of activities can help to keep your exercise routine interesting and challenging.
5. Flexibility: Life is unpredictable, and finding an exercise routine that is flexible and adaptable can help you to maintain your exercise habit even when your schedule or circumstances change.
6. Mental health: Exercise can have significant benefits for mental health, including reducing stress and improving mood. Finding an exercise routine that works for you can help you to experience these benefits and support your overall well-being.

Overall, finding an exercise routine that works for you is essential for creating a sustainable exercise habit that supports your physical and mental health. By considering your individual needs, preferences, and circumstances, you can find an exercise routine that you enjoy and that fits into your lifestyle, making it more likely that you'll stick with it and reap the benefits.

- **Different types of exercise and their benefits**

There are several different types of exercise, each with its own benefits. Here are some of the most common types of exercise and their benefits:

1. Aerobic exercise: Aerobic exercise, also known as cardio, is any type of exercise that increases your heart rate and breathing. Examples include running, cycling, swimming, and dancing. Benefits of aerobic exercise include improved cardiovascular health, increased endurance, and weight management.
2. Strength training: Strength training involves using weights, resistance bands, or your own body weight to build muscle strength and endurance. Benefits of strength training include improved muscle tone and definition, increased metabolism, and better bone health.
3. Flexibility exercises: Flexibility exercises, such as stretching, yoga, and Pilates, help to improve flexibility and range of motion. Benefits of flexibility exercises include improved posture, reduced risk of injury, and decreased muscle soreness.
4. Balance exercises: Balance exercises help to improve balance and stability, which can reduce the risk of falls and injuries. Examples include standing on one leg, yoga, and tai chi.
5. High-intensity interval training (HIIT): HIIT involves short bursts of high-intensity exercise followed by periods of rest or lower-intensity exercise. Benefits of HIIT include improved cardiovascular health, increased calorie burn, and improved endurance.

6. Low-impact exercises: Low-impact exercises, such as swimming, cycling, and walking, are gentler on the joints and can be beneficial for people with joint pain or injuries. Benefits of low-impact exercises include improved cardiovascular health, weight management, and reduced risk of injury.

Overall, incorporating a variety of types of exercise into your routine can help you to achieve a range of benefits for your physical and mental health. By choosing activities that you enjoy and that fit your individual needs and preferences, you can create a sustainable exercise habit that supports your overall well-being.

- **How to choose an exercise program that fits your lifestyle and preferences**

Choosing an exercise program that fits your lifestyle and preferences is important for creating a sustainable and enjoyable exercise habit. Here are some steps you can take to choose an exercise program that works for you:

1. Consider your goals: What do you want to achieve with exercise? Do you want to improve your cardiovascular health, build muscle, lose weight, or reduce stress? Your goals can help to guide you in choosing an exercise program that is tailored to your specific needs and preferences.
2. Assess your fitness level: Consider your current fitness level and any limitations or health concerns you may have. If you're new to exercise or have health concerns, you may want to start with a low-impact program or consult with a healthcare professional or certified fitness trainer.
3. Determine your availability: How much time do you have to devote to exercise? Consider your schedule and other commitments when choosing an exercise program. If you have limited time, you may want to choose a program that offers shorter workouts or that you can do at home.
4. Explore your options: There are many different types of exercise programs, from group fitness classes to personal training to online programs. Explore different options and consider what appeals to you, such as group exercise classes, outdoor activities, or solo workouts.
5. Consider your preferences: What activities do you enjoy? If you enjoy dancing, for example, you may want to try a dance fitness class. If you prefer outdoor activities, you may want to consider hiking, cycling, or running. Choosing activities that you enjoy can help to make exercise more enjoyable and sustainable.
6. Plan for variety: Incorporating a variety of activities into your exercise program can help to keep things interesting and challenging. Consider mixing up your workouts, such as doing strength training on some days and cardio on others.
7. Listen to your body: Pay attention to how your body feels during and after exercise. If you experience pain or discomfort, modify or adjust your program as needed.

By considering your goals, fitness level, availability, preferences, and variety, you can choose an exercise program that works for your lifestyle and supports your overall health and well-being. Remember to be flexible and adaptable as your needs and preferences change over time.

IV. The Power of Consistency

- **Incorporating exercise into your daily routine**

Incorporating exercise into your daily routine can be an effective way to make physical activity a regular and sustainable habit. Here are some tips for incorporating exercise into your daily routine:

1. Schedule it in: Treat exercise like any other appointment or commitment by scheduling it into your calendar. Set aside specific times each week for exercise and prioritize these appointments like you would with other important commitments.
2. Make it convenient: Choose exercise activities that are convenient and easily accessible to you. This might mean finding a gym or fitness center near your home or workplace, or taking a walk or jog around your neighborhood.
3. Start small: If you're new to exercise, start with small goals and gradually build up your intensity and duration over time. This can help you to avoid injury and burnout, and can make exercise feel less overwhelming.
4. Multitask: Look for ways to incorporate exercise into other daily activities. For example, you might try walking or cycling to work, taking a walk during your lunch break, or doing bodyweight exercises while watching TV.
5. Find an accountability partner: Having a friend, family member, or colleague to exercise with can provide motivation and accountability. You might also consider hiring a personal trainer or joining a fitness class or group.
6. Take breaks and stretch: If you have a sedentary job or spend a lot of time sitting, take regular breaks to stretch or move around. Consider standing or walking while on the phone, taking the stairs instead of the elevator, or doing some quick stretches at your desk.
7. Make it fun: Choose exercise activities that you enjoy and that feel like fun rather than a chore. This can help to make exercise more sustainable and enjoyable over time.

By incorporating exercise into your daily routine, you can make physical activity a regular and sustainable habit that supports your overall health and well-being. Remember to be patient with yourself and celebrate your progress along the way.

- **Tips for making exercise a regular habit**

Making exercise a regular habit can be challenging, but it is key to reaping the benefits of physical activity. Here are some tips for making exercise a regular habit:

1. Set achievable goals: Setting specific, achievable goals can help to keep you motivated and on track. Start with small goals and gradually increase your intensity and duration over time.
2. Schedule it in: Treat exercise like any other appointment or commitment by scheduling it into your calendar. Set aside specific times each week for exercise and prioritize these appointments like you would with other important commitments.
3. Find an accountability partner: Having a friend, family member, or colleague to exercise with can provide motivation and accountability. You might also consider hiring a personal trainer or joining a fitness class or group.
4. Start small: If you're new to exercise, start with small goals and gradually build up your intensity and duration over time. This can help you to avoid injury and burnout, and can make exercise feel less overwhelming.
5. Choose activities you enjoy: Exercise shouldn't feel like a chore. Choose activities that you enjoy and that feel like fun rather than a burden. This can help to make exercise more sustainable and enjoyable over time.
6. Make it a habit: Consistency is key to making exercise a regular habit. Try to exercise at the same time each day, or on the same days each week, to help establish a routine.
7. Track your progress: Keeping track of your progress can help to keep you motivated and focused. Consider tracking your workouts, measuring your fitness levels, or taking before-and-after photos to monitor your progress over time.
8. Celebrate your successes: Celebrate your successes, no matter how small. Whether you've completed a new workout, hit a new personal best, or simply made it to your scheduled exercise sessions for the week, take time to recognize your accomplishments and reward yourself for your efforts.

By following these tips and making exercise a regular part of your routine, you can reap the many benefits of physical activity and improve your overall health and well-being.

- **The benefits of consistency in exercise**

Consistency in exercise is crucial for achieving and maintaining a healthy and active lifestyle. Here are some of the benefits of consistency in exercise:

1. Improved fitness: Consistently exercising helps to improve your overall fitness levels, including your cardiovascular health, muscle strength, and flexibility. As you exercise regularly, your body adapts and becomes better at performing physical activity, allowing you to gradually increase your intensity and duration.
2. Weight management: Consistently exercising can help with weight management by burning calories and building muscle mass. Regular exercise can also help to boost your metabolism, which can help you to burn more calories throughout the day.
3. Reduced risk of chronic disease: Consistent exercise has been shown to reduce the risk of chronic diseases such as heart disease, diabetes, and certain types of cancer.

Physical activity helps to improve blood pressure, cholesterol levels, and insulin sensitivity, all of which are important for maintaining good health.

4. Improved mental health: Exercise has been shown to have numerous benefits for mental health, including reducing stress and anxiety, improving mood, and boosting self-esteem. Consistent exercise can help to establish a routine that supports your mental health and provides a positive outlet for stress and emotions.
5. Increased energy and productivity: Consistent exercise can help to boost your energy levels and improve your focus and productivity. Exercise releases endorphins, which can help to reduce feelings of fatigue and increase feelings of alertness and well-being.

By being consistent with your exercise routine, you can reap these benefits and achieve your fitness and health goals. Consistency doesn't mean you have to exercise intensely every day, but rather that you establish a routine that works for you and stick to it over time. This can help to make exercise a regular and sustainable part of your lifestyle.

V. Mastering Fitness

- **Setting realistic goals for exercise**

Setting realistic goals for exercise is an important part of establishing a sustainable exercise routine. Here are some tips for setting realistic exercise goals:

1. Start small: If you're new to exercise or haven't exercised in a while, start with small goals and gradually increase your intensity and duration over time. This can help to avoid injury and burnout, and can make exercise feel less overwhelming.
2. Be specific: Set specific, measurable goals that are tailored to your individual needs and preferences. For example, instead of setting a goal to "exercise more," set a goal to "exercise for 30 minutes, 3 times per week."
3. Consider your schedule: When setting exercise goals, consider your schedule and other commitments. Make sure your goals are achievable within your existing routine, and consider whether you need to adjust your schedule to make exercise a priority.
4. Be realistic: Set goals that are challenging but achievable. Don't set yourself up for failure by setting unrealistic goals that are too difficult or time-consuming.
5. Be flexible: Be prepared to adjust your goals as needed. Life can be unpredictable, and it's important to be flexible and adapt your goals as circumstances change.
6. Celebrate your successes: Celebrate your successes, no matter how small. Recognize your accomplishments and reward yourself for your efforts. This can help to keep you motivated and focused on achieving your goals.

By setting realistic exercise goals, you can establish a sustainable exercise routine and achieve your fitness and health goals over time. Remember that consistency is key, and that making small, incremental changes can add up to significant improvements in your fitness and overall health.

- **The importance of tracking progress**

Tracking your progress is an important part of achieving your fitness and health goals. Here are some reasons why tracking your progress is important:

1. Motivation: Tracking your progress can help to keep you motivated and focused on your goals. When you see progress over time, it can help to reinforce the benefits of exercise and encourage you to continue.
2. Accountability: Tracking your progress can help to hold you accountable to your goals. When you see that you're not making progress, it can be a sign that you need to make changes to your routine or re-evaluate your goals.
3. Identification of trends and patterns: By tracking your progress over time, you can identify trends and patterns in your performance. This can help you to make adjustments to your routine and optimize your progress.
4. Feedback: Tracking your progress can provide valuable feedback on your performance. By analyzing your progress, you can identify areas where you're excelling and areas where you need to improve.
5. Measurement of success: Tracking your progress can help you to measure your success and celebrate your accomplishments. This can help to reinforce the benefits of exercise and encourage you to continue.

There are many ways to track your progress, including keeping a workout journal, using a fitness app, or working with a personal trainer. Whatever method you choose, make sure it's something that works for you and that you're consistent in tracking your progress over time. By tracking your progress, you can achieve your fitness and health goals and establish a sustainable exercise routine that supports your overall well-being.

- **How to stay motivated and overcome obstacles**

Staying motivated and overcoming obstacles is an important part of maintaining a consistent exercise routine. Here are some tips to help you stay motivated and overcome obstacles:

1. Set realistic goals: Setting realistic goals can help to keep you motivated and focused on your progress. Make sure your goals are achievable and tailored to your individual needs and preferences.
2. Find a workout buddy: Working out with a friend or family member can provide motivation and accountability. It can also make exercise more enjoyable and fun.
3. Mix up your routine: Trying new exercises and activities can help to prevent boredom and keep you engaged in your routine. Mix up your routine by trying different types of exercise or adding variety to your workouts.
4. Keep a positive attitude: Maintaining a positive attitude can help to overcome obstacles and challenges. Focus on your progress and accomplishments, and don't get discouraged by setbacks or setbacks.

5. Plan ahead: Planning your workouts in advance can help to ensure that you stay on track with your routine. Make sure you have everything you need for your workouts, and schedule your workouts around your other commitments.
6. Reward yourself: Celebrate your accomplishments and reward yourself for your hard work. This can help to reinforce the benefits of exercise and encourage you to continue.
7. Seek support: If you're struggling to stay motivated or overcome obstacles, seek support from friends, family, or a professional. A personal trainer or fitness coach can provide guidance and accountability, and can help you to stay on track with your goals.

By staying motivated and overcoming obstacles, you can establish a sustainable exercise routine that supports your overall health and well-being. Remember that consistency is key, and that making small, incremental changes can add up to significant improvements over time.

VI. A Holistic Approach to Weight Loss

- **Combining exercise with a healthy diet plan for maximum weight loss**

Combining exercise with a healthy diet plan is an effective way to achieve maximum weight loss. Here are some reasons why:

1. Calorie deficit: To lose weight, you need to create a calorie deficit, which means burning more calories than you consume. Exercise helps to burn calories and increase your metabolism, while a healthy diet plan provides the nutrients and energy you need to fuel your workouts and support your overall health.
2. Muscle building: Exercise, particularly resistance training, can help to build muscle, which increases your metabolism and helps to burn more calories at rest. A healthy diet plan that includes adequate protein and nutrients can support muscle growth and repair.
3. Improved energy and mood: Regular exercise and a healthy diet plan can improve your energy levels and mood, helping you to stay motivated and focused on your goals.
4. Reduced risk of chronic diseases: Regular exercise and a healthy diet plan can help to reduce the risk of chronic diseases, such as obesity, heart disease, and diabetes.

To combine exercise with a healthy diet plan for maximum weight loss, consider the following tips:

1. Choose whole, nutrient-dense foods: Focus on eating whole, nutrient-dense foods, such as fruits, vegetables, lean proteins, and whole grains. These foods provide the

nutrients and energy you need to support your workouts and help you feel full and satisfied.
2. Avoid processed foods: Avoid processed and high-calorie foods, such as sugary snacks, fast food, and processed meats. These foods are often high in calories and low in nutrients, and can sabotage your weight loss efforts.
3. Stay hydrated: Drink plenty of water to stay hydrated and support your workouts. Avoid sugary drinks and alcohol, which can add extra calories to your diet.
4. Plan your meals and workouts: Plan your meals and workouts in advance to help you stay on track with your goals. Make sure you have healthy snacks on hand for when you need a quick boost of energy.
5. Consult with a professional: Consider working with a nutritionist or personal trainer to develop a customized plan that meets your individual needs and preferences.

By combining exercise with a healthy diet plan, you can achieve maximum weight loss and improve your overall health and well-being. Remember to be patient and consistent, and focus on making small, sustainable changes to your lifestyle over time.

- **How exercise and diet work together to achieve weight loss goals**

Exercise and diet are both important components of a weight loss program, and work together to help achieve weight loss goals in several ways:

1. Calorie deficit: To lose weight, you need to create a calorie deficit, which means burning more calories than you consume. Exercise helps to burn calories, while a healthy diet provides the nutrients and energy you need to support your workouts and support your overall health.
2. Muscle building: Exercise, particularly resistance training, can help to build muscle, which increases your metabolism and helps to burn more calories at rest. A healthy diet plan that includes adequate protein and nutrients can support muscle growth and repair.
3. Improved energy and mood: Regular exercise and a healthy diet plan can improve your energy levels and mood, helping you to stay motivated and focused on your weight loss goals.
4. Reduced risk of chronic diseases: Regular exercise and a healthy diet plan can help to reduce the risk of chronic diseases, such as obesity, heart disease, and diabetes.

To achieve weight loss goals, it is important to combine exercise and diet in a balanced and sustainable way. Here are some tips for combining exercise and diet for weight loss:

1. Create a calorie deficit: Use a combination of exercise and diet to create a calorie deficit, which means burning more calories than you consume. Aim to lose 1-2 pounds per week, which is a safe and sustainable rate of weight loss.

2. Choose whole, nutrient-dense foods: Focus on eating whole, nutrient-dense foods, such as fruits, vegetables, lean proteins, and whole grains. These foods provide the nutrients and energy you need to support your workouts and help you feel full and satisfied.
3. Avoid processed foods: Avoid processed and high-calorie foods, such as sugary snacks, fast food, and processed meats. These foods are often high in calories and low in nutrients, and can sabotage your weight loss efforts.
4. Exercise regularly: Aim for at least 150 minutes of moderate-intensity exercise per week, such as brisk walking, cycling, or swimming. Include both aerobic and resistance training to burn calories and build muscle.
5. Stay hydrated: Drink plenty of water to stay hydrated and support your workouts. Avoid sugary drinks and alcohol, which can add extra calories to your diet.

By combining exercise and diet, you can achieve weight loss goals and improve your overall health and well-being. Remember to be patient and consistent, and focus on making small, sustainable changes to your lifestyle over time.

- **The benefits of a comprehensive weight loss plan**

A comprehensive weight loss plan is a plan that combines multiple strategies and approaches to help you lose weight in a healthy and sustainable way. Such a plan can offer many benefits, including:

1. Improved overall health: A comprehensive weight loss plan can improve your overall health and reduce the risk of chronic diseases such as heart disease, diabetes, and high blood pressure.
2. Increased energy levels: Regular exercise and a healthy diet can help to increase your energy levels, allowing you to feel more alert and productive throughout the day.
3. Better sleep quality: Regular exercise and a healthy diet can help to improve sleep quality, allowing you to feel more rested and refreshed each morning.
4. Sustainable weight loss: By combining different strategies, such as a healthy diet, regular exercise, and behavioral changes, a comprehensive weight loss plan can help you achieve sustainable weight loss and maintain a healthy weight in the long term.
5. Improved self-esteem and body image: Losing weight can help to improve your self-esteem and body image, which can have a positive impact on your mental health and well-being.
6. Reduced stress levels: Exercise and healthy eating can help to reduce stress levels and improve your overall mood and sense of well-being.
7. Increased social support: Joining a weight loss program or working with a personal trainer can provide social support and motivation, making it easier to stick to your weight loss goals.

Overall, a comprehensive weight loss plan can offer numerous benefits for both your physical and mental health. By combining different strategies and approaches, you can achieve sustainable weight loss and improve your overall well-being.

CHAPTER 5

Managing Stress and Getting Enough Sleep

I. Introduction

- Importance of managing stress and getting enough sleep for overall well-being

II. Effects of Chronic Stress on Health

- Physical health problems associated with chronic stress
- Mental health problems associated with chronic stress

III. Importance of Sleep for Health

- Effects of chronic sleep deprivation on health
- Importance of sleep for brain function, memory consolidation, and physical restoration

IV. Strategies for Managing Stress and Improving Sleep

- Stress-reducing activities such as meditation and deep breathing exercises
- Establishing a regular sleep schedule and creating a sleep-conducive environment

I. Introduction

Stress and lack of sleep have become increasingly common in our modern lives, with many people facing constant demands from work, family, and social obligations. However, these factors can have significant negative impacts on our health and well-being, making it important to prioritize stress management and healthy sleep habits. While many people focus on exercise and nutrition to improve their physical health, the importance of stress management and sleep cannot be overstated.

Chronic stress has been linked to a range of physical and mental health problems, including high blood pressure, heart disease, obesity, anxiety, and depression. In addition, sleep deprivation has been shown to have detrimental effects on cognitive function, mood, and overall health. By incorporating stress-reducing activities and healthy sleep habits into our daily routine, we can improve our physical and mental health, reduce the risk of chronic health problems, and increase our overall well-being.

In this chapter, we will explore the importance of managing stress and getting enough sleep, and provide strategies for incorporating stress-reducing activities and healthy sleep habits into our daily routine. We will also discuss the benefits of making these changes, and provide resources for individuals who are looking to improve their stress management and sleep habits.

- **Importance of managing stress and getting enough sleep for overall well-being**

Managing stress and getting enough sleep are crucial for overall well-being. Stress is a natural response to challenging situations, but chronic stress can have negative impacts on our physical and mental health, leading to a range of health problems such as high blood pressure, heart disease, obesity, anxiety, and depression. Chronic stress can also impair our immune system, making us more susceptible to illness and disease.

Getting enough sleep is equally important for our well-being. Sleep is a critical process that allows our body to rest, recover and repair itself. Chronic sleep deprivation has been linked to a range of negative health outcomes, including obesity, diabetes, high blood pressure, heart disease, and impaired cognitive function.

When we manage stress and get enough sleep, we are able to reduce our risk of developing these health problems and increase our overall well-being. By reducing stress, we can improve our mental health, reduce our risk of chronic disease, and enhance our ability to cope with life's challenges. Getting enough sleep allows us to feel more energized, improve our cognitive function, and reduce our risk of health problems associated with sleep deprivation.

In summary, managing stress and getting enough sleep are important for overall well-being. By prioritizing stress management and healthy sleep habits, we can improve our physical and mental health, reduce our risk of chronic disease, and increase our overall quality of life.

II. Effects of Chronic Stress on Health

- **Physical health problems associated with chronic stress**

Chronic stress can have numerous negative effects on physical health. When the body is exposed to prolonged periods of stress, it activates the sympathetic nervous system, leading to the release of stress hormones such as cortisol and adrenaline. Over time, the constant presence of these hormones can have detrimental effects on the body, leading to a range of physical health problems, including:

1. High blood pressure: Chronic stress can increase blood pressure levels, increasing the risk of heart disease, stroke, and kidney damage.
2. Cardiovascular disease: Chronic stress can cause inflammation and damage to blood vessels, leading to the development of cardiovascular disease.
3. Obesity: Stress can trigger overeating or unhealthy eating habits, leading to weight gain and obesity.
4. Diabetes: Chronic stress can lead to elevated blood sugar levels and insulin resistance, increasing the risk of developing type 2 diabetes.
5. Immune system dysfunction: Chronic stress can impair the immune system, making it more difficult for the body to fight off infections and illnesses.
6. Digestive problems: Stress can cause digestive issues such as irritable bowel syndrome (IBS), acid reflux, and ulcers.
7. Sleep disturbances: Chronic stress can disrupt sleep patterns, leading to sleep deprivation and a range of negative health consequences.

These are just some of the physical health problems associated with chronic stress. It is important to prioritize stress management and seek help if you are experiencing chronic stress or stress-related health problems.

- **Mental health problems associated with chronic stress**

Chronic stress can also have negative effects on our mental health. When we experience stress, it can trigger a range of emotional and cognitive responses that can impact our mental well-being. Here are some of the mental health problems associated with chronic stress:

1. Anxiety: Chronic stress can lead to anxiety, which is characterized by excessive worry, fear, and apprehension.

2. Depression: Chronic stress can also lead to depression, which is characterized by feelings of sadness, hopelessness, and low self-esteem.
3. Post-traumatic stress disorder (PTSD): People who experience traumatic events may develop PTSD, a mental health disorder that is characterized by flashbacks, nightmares, and severe anxiety.
4. Substance abuse: People may turn to drugs or alcohol to cope with chronic stress, leading to addiction and substance abuse problems.
5. Burnout: Chronic stress can lead to burnout, a state of emotional, physical, and mental exhaustion that can result from long-term exposure to stressors.
6. Insomnia: Chronic stress can also cause sleep disturbances, leading to insomnia and other sleep disorders.

These are just a few of the mental health problems associated with chronic stress. It is important to prioritize stress management and seek help if you are experiencing chronic stress or stress-related mental health problems. Counseling, therapy, and other stress management techniques can help individuals better cope with stress and improve their mental health.

III. Importance of Sleep for Health

- **Effects of chronic sleep deprivation on health**

Chronic sleep deprivation occurs when an individual consistently fails to get enough sleep over a prolonged period of time. This can have a range of negative effects on physical and mental health. Here are some of the effects of chronic sleep deprivation on health:

1. Increased risk of chronic diseases: Chronic sleep deprivation is associated with an increased risk of developing chronic diseases such as diabetes, heart disease, and obesity.
2. Impaired cognitive function: Sleep is essential for brain function, and chronic sleep deprivation can impair cognitive function, including memory, concentration, and decision-making.
3. Weakened immune system: Sleep is crucial for immune function, and chronic sleep deprivation can weaken the immune system, making individuals more susceptible to infections and illnesses.
4. Mood disturbances: Chronic sleep deprivation can lead to mood disturbances, including irritability, anxiety, and depression.
5. Weight gain: Chronic sleep deprivation can disrupt the hormones that regulate appetite, leading to overeating and weight gain.
6. Increased risk of accidents: Chronic sleep deprivation can impair reaction time and decision-making, increasing the risk of accidents.
7. Increased risk of mortality: Chronic sleep deprivation has been associated with an increased risk of mortality, particularly from cardiovascular disease.

These are just some of the negative effects of chronic sleep deprivation on health. It is important to prioritize getting enough sleep and seek help if you are experiencing chronic sleep problems. Sleep hygiene practices, such as establishing a regular sleep schedule and creating a comfortable sleep environment, can help individuals improve their sleep habits and overall health.

- **Importance of sleep for brain function, memory consolidation, and physical restoration**

Sleep is essential for many aspects of physical and mental health, including brain function, memory consolidation, and physical restoration. Here are some of the key reasons why sleep is important:

1. Brain function: Sleep is crucial for brain function. During sleep, the brain consolidates memories and processes information from the previous day, which helps to improve cognitive function and overall brain performance.
2. Memory consolidation: Sleep plays an important role in memory consolidation, which is the process by which the brain converts short-term memories into long-term memories. This process is important for learning and retaining new information.
3. Physical restoration: Sleep is also important for physical restoration, including muscle repair and growth, and the release of hormones that regulate appetite, metabolism, and energy.
4. Mood regulation: Sleep is essential for regulating mood and emotional well-being. Chronic sleep deprivation has been linked to an increased risk of mood disorders such as depression and anxiety.
5. Immune system function: Sleep is important for the proper functioning of the immune system, which helps to protect the body against infections and disease.

Overall, sleep plays a vital role in many aspects of physical and mental health, and getting enough quality sleep is essential for overall well-being. Experts recommend that adults aim for 7-9 hours of sleep per night, although individual needs may vary. It is important to prioritize good sleep habits and seek help if you are experiencing chronic sleep problems.

IV. Strategies for Managing Stress and Improving Sleep

- **Stress-reducing activities such as meditation and deep breathing exercises**

Stress can have a negative impact on physical and mental health, but there are many stress-reducing activities that can help promote relaxation and well-being. Here are some examples:

1. Meditation: Meditation involves focusing your attention and being present in the moment, which can help reduce stress and promote a sense of calm. There are many different types of meditation, including mindfulness meditation, which involves paying attention to your breath and physical sensations in the present moment.
2. Deep breathing exercises: Deep breathing exercises involve taking slow, deep breaths and exhaling slowly. This can help calm the nervous system and reduce feelings of stress and anxiety.
3. Mindfulness practices: Mindfulness practices involve focusing your attention on the present moment and observing your thoughts and feelings without judgment. This can help reduce stress and promote a sense of calm.
4. Exercise: Exercise is a natural stress reducer that can help improve mood and reduce feelings of anxiety and depression.

Overall, there are many different stress-reducing activities that can be incorporated into a daily routine to promote relaxation and well-being. It is important to find activities that work for you and to prioritize self-care and stress reduction as part of a healthy lifestyle.

- **Establishing a regular sleep schedule and creating a sleep-conducive environment**

Establishing a regular sleep schedule and creating a sleep-conducive environment are important steps in promoting healthy sleep habits. Here are some tips:

1. Stick to a regular sleep schedule: Try to go to bed and wake up at the same time every day, even on weekends. This can help regulate your body's internal clock and improve the quality of your sleep.
2. Create a sleep-conducive environment: Make sure your bedroom is dark, quiet, and cool, with comfortable bedding and a supportive mattress. Consider using blackout curtains or a white noise machine to block out light and noise.
3. Limit screen time before bed: The blue light emitted by electronic devices can interfere with sleep. Try to avoid using electronic devices for at least an hour before bed.
4. Avoid caffeine and alcohol: Caffeine and alcohol can interfere with sleep quality. Try to limit your intake of these substances, especially in the hours before bedtime.
5. Practice relaxation techniques: Relaxation techniques, such as deep breathing exercises, progressive muscle relaxation, or guided imagery, can help calm the mind and prepare the body for sleep.

By establishing a regular sleep schedule and creating a sleep-conducive environment, you can improve the quality of your sleep and promote overall health and well-being. It is important to prioritize good sleep habits as part of a healthy lifestyle.

<h1>CHAPTER 6</h1>

<h2>Staying Motivated and Overcoming Obstacles</h2>

I. Introduction

- The importance of staying motivated to achieve fitness goals
- Overcoming obstacles that may arise during the journey to better health and fitness

II. Key Strategies for Achieving Realistic Fitness Goals

- Setting realistic goals and expectations for yourself
- Breaking down larger goals into smaller, more manageable steps
- Focusing on progress rather than perfection

III. Strategies for making exercise a regular and enjoyable part of your lifestyle

- Finding an exercise routine that you enjoy and look forward to
- Varying your workouts to prevent boredom and maintain interest
- Incorporating exercise into your daily routine

IV. Strategies for Staying Motivated and Overcoming Obstacles in Your Fitness Journey

- Staying accountable by tracking progress and celebrating successes
- Seeking support from friends, family, or a professional coach
- Overcoming common obstacles, such as lack of time, motivation, or energy

V. Key Components of a Sustainable Fitness Routine

- Recognizing the importance of rest and recovery in preventing burnout
- Incorporating mindfulness practices, such as meditation or deep breathing, into your routine to reduce stress and increase focus
- Adjusting your approach as needed, and being willing to try new things to keep yourself engaged and motivated

I. Introduction

Staying motivated to achieve fitness goals can be challenging, especially when faced with obstacles such as lack of time, energy, or resources. However, it is important to recognize that making positive changes to your health and fitness can have a significant impact on your overall well-being.

In this chapter, we will explore various strategies for staying motivated and overcoming obstacles that may arise during your journey to better health and fitness. From setting realistic goals and finding an exercise routine that works for you, to staying accountable and seeking support from others, we will provide tips and insights to help you stay on track and achieve your goals.

We will also discuss the importance of rest and recovery in preventing burnout, as well as the benefits of incorporating mindfulness practices into your routine to reduce stress and increase focus. By the end of this chapter, you will have a range of strategies at your disposal for staying motivated and overcoming obstacles, no matter where you are in your fitness journey.

- **The importance of staying motivated to achieve fitness goals**

Staying motivated is crucial for achieving fitness goals because it provides the drive and energy needed to make consistent progress. Without motivation, it can be easy to fall into old habits or give up when faced with obstacles or setbacks.

Motivation helps to keep individuals focused on their goals and reminds them of the reasons why they started on their fitness journey in the first place. It also provides a sense of accomplishment and satisfaction when goals are achieved, which can in turn help to boost motivation further.

Furthermore, staying motivated is important for maintaining a positive mindset and developing a sense of self-efficacy. When individuals are able to achieve their fitness goals through consistent effort and dedication, it can lead to increased confidence and a belief in one's ability to overcome challenges in other areas of life.

Overall, staying motivated is key to achieving and maintaining a healthy lifestyle, and it requires a combination of intrinsic and extrinsic motivation, as well as ongoing effort and commitment.

- **Overcoming obstacles that may arise during the journey to better health and fitness**

Achieving better health and fitness can be a challenging journey, and there are many obstacles that may arise along the way. These obstacles can take many different forms, such as injuries, illnesses, lack of time, lack of support from others, or simply feeling unmotivated or discouraged.

It's important to recognize that obstacles are a normal part of any journey, and that it's possible to overcome them with the right mindset and strategies. One effective strategy for overcoming obstacles is to develop a plan or strategy ahead of time for how to handle challenges when they arise. This may involve creating backup workout plans for days when time is tight, seeking out support from friends or family members, or finding alternative forms of exercise when injuries occur.

Another strategy for overcoming obstacles is to stay focused on the end goal and remind yourself of the reasons why you started on your fitness journey in the first place. It can also be helpful to celebrate small victories along the way, as this can help to boost motivation and provide a sense of accomplishment.

Finally, it's important to remember that setbacks and obstacles are a normal part of the process, and that it's okay to take a break or adjust your goals if needed. The key is to stay flexible, maintain a positive attitude, and keep moving forward towards better health and fitness.

II. Key Strategies for Achieving Realistic Fitness Goals

- **Setting realistic goals and expectations for yourself**

Setting realistic goals and expectations for yourself is an important aspect of achieving and maintaining success in any fitness journey. When you set unrealistic goals or expect immediate results, it can lead to disappointment, frustration, and ultimately, giving up on your goals.

Instead, it's important to set achievable goals that are specific, measurable, and time-bound. For example, instead of setting a vague goal like "lose weight," a more specific and measurable goal could be to "lose 10 pounds in 8 weeks by exercising 3 times per week and following a healthy diet."

It's also important to be realistic about the time and effort it will take to achieve your goals. Sustainable changes take time and consistent effort, so it's important to be patient and not get discouraged if you don't see immediate results.

In addition, it's important to focus on progress rather than perfection. Celebrate small successes along the way and recognize that setbacks and challenges are a normal part of any journey. By setting realistic goals and expectations for yourself, you can stay motivated and focused on achieving long-term success in your fitness journey.

- **Breaking down larger goals into smaller, more manageable steps**

Breaking down larger goals into smaller, more manageable steps is an effective strategy for achieving success in any fitness journey. When you have a large, long-term goal, it can feel overwhelming and difficult to know where to start. By breaking it down into smaller, more achievable steps, you can create a clear roadmap to follow and make steady progress towards your ultimate goal.

For example, if your long-term goal is to run a marathon, you can break it down into smaller, more manageable steps such as:

1. Start by running for 20-30 minutes at a time, 3-4 times per week.
2. Increase your running time gradually each week, adding 5-10 minutes at a time.
3. Incorporate strength training and stretching into your routine to prevent injuries and improve performance.
4. Sign up for a 5k or 10k race as a stepping stone towards the marathon.
5. Follow a training plan specifically designed for marathon preparation.
6. Focus on proper nutrition and hydration to support your training and recovery.

By breaking down your larger goal into smaller, achievable steps, you can create a sense of accomplishment and momentum as you make progress towards your ultimate goal. It can also help you to stay motivated and focused on your journey, rather than feeling overwhelmed by the bigger picture.

- **Focusing on progress rather than perfection**

Focusing on progress rather than perfection is an important aspect of setting realistic goals and maintaining motivation. It is important to acknowledge that progress is not always linear, and setbacks may occur along the way. Rather than being discouraged by setbacks or failures, it is important to recognize them as opportunities for learning and growth.

To focus on progress rather than perfection, it can be helpful to track your progress and celebrate small victories. For example, if your goal is to run a 5K race, celebrating completing a 1-mile run without stopping or improving your time by even a few seconds can help keep you motivated and focused on the bigger goal.

It is also important to have patience and understand that achieving long-term goals takes time and consistency. It can be helpful to break down larger goals into smaller, more manageable steps and focus on making progress in those smaller steps. This can help you build momentum and confidence as you work toward your larger goal.

By setting realistic goals and focusing on progress rather than perfection, you can maintain motivation and overcome obstacles on your journey to better health and fitness.

III. Strategies for making exercise a regular and enjoyable part of your lifestyle

- **Finding an exercise routine that you enjoy and look forward to**

Finding an exercise routine that you enjoy and look forward to can make a significant difference in your motivation to stay active. It's important to choose activities that you find enjoyable and engaging, so you're more likely to stick with them in the long run. This could be anything from running, cycling, or swimming, to dancing, yoga, or martial arts. There are countless options available, so take the time to explore different activities and find the ones that resonate with you.

When you find an exercise routine that you enjoy, you're more likely to look forward to it and feel motivated to stick with it. Additionally, finding a routine that you can do with others, like a group fitness class or sports team, can help keep you accountable and make the experience more enjoyable. By focusing on activities that you genuinely enjoy, you can make exercise a regular and sustainable part of your lifestyle.

- **Varying your workouts to prevent boredom and maintain interest**

Varying your workouts can help prevent boredom and maintain your interest in exercise. Doing the same routine day after day can become monotonous and lead to burnout. By incorporating different types of exercises or activities, you can challenge your body in new ways and keep things fresh and interesting. This can also prevent plateaus in your progress, as your body adapts to the same workout routine over time.

For example, if you typically go for a run every day, consider adding in some strength training or yoga on alternate days. If you enjoy group fitness classes, try out different formats like spinning, dance cardio, or kickboxing. You can also switch up the intensity of your workouts, alternating between high-intensity interval training (HIIT) and lower-intensity steady-state cardio.

Varying your workouts can also help prevent injuries by giving your muscles and joints a break from repetitive movements. It can also challenge your mind and prevent exercise from feeling like a chore. By finding different activities that you enjoy, you may also be more likely to stick with your exercise routine long-term.

- **Incorporating exercise into your daily routine**

Regular exercise is an important component of a healthy lifestyle, but finding the time and motivation to work out can be a challenge. One way to overcome this obstacle is to incorporate exercise into your daily routine. By making physical activity a regular part of your daily life, you can improve your fitness level, boost your energy, and reduce your risk of chronic diseases.

There are several ways to incorporate exercise into your daily routine, depending on your preferences and lifestyle. For example, you could:

- Walk or bike to work, school, or errands instead of driving or taking public transportation
- Take the stairs instead of the elevator
- Schedule regular exercise breaks throughout the day, such as a morning walk or lunchtime yoga class
- Use household chores as an opportunity to increase your activity level, such as by doing a few squats or lunges while vacuuming or mopping
- Make social events active, such as by going for a hike with friends instead of meeting for drinks

Incorporating exercise into your daily routine can help you establish a consistent exercise habit, which can be beneficial for long-term health and fitness. It can also make exercise feel more natural and enjoyable, as it becomes a regular part of your day-to-day life.

IV. Strategies for Staying Motivated and Overcoming Obstacles in Your Fitness Journey

- **Staying accountable by tracking progress and celebrating successes**

Staying accountable and tracking your progress is an essential part of staying motivated and overcoming obstacles on the journey to better health and fitness. One effective way to do this is by keeping a record of your workouts, such as a fitness journal or mobile app. This can help you monitor your progress over time and identify areas where you may need to make adjustments to your routine.

Additionally, celebrating your successes along the way, no matter how small, can help keep you motivated and focused on your goals. This can be as simple as acknowledging and rewarding yourself for consistently sticking to your workout schedule or reaching a new personal record in your exercise routine. It's important to remember that progress is not always linear, and setbacks may occur. However, staying positive and focusing on the successes and progress made can help keep you motivated and on track towards achieving your fitness goals.

- **Seeking support from friends, family, or a professional coach**

Seeking support from friends, family, or a professional coach can be a powerful tool in staying motivated and overcoming obstacles. Having a support system can provide encouragement, accountability, and guidance, which can make a significant difference in achieving fitness goals. Friends and family can provide emotional support, offer to exercise together, and be a source of motivation. A professional coach or personal trainer can provide personalized guidance and support, help create a customized workout plan, and hold you accountable for your progress. It can also be helpful to join a fitness community or group to connect with others who share similar goals and experiences. This can provide additional support and motivation, as well as a sense of belonging and community. Ultimately, seeking support can help you stay on track and make progress towards your fitness goals.

- **Overcoming common obstacles, such as lack of time, motivation, or energy**

Overcoming obstacles is an essential part of achieving fitness goals. Common obstacles can include a lack of time, motivation, or energy. It's important to recognize these challenges and develop strategies to overcome them.

One effective strategy for overcoming time constraints is to schedule workouts into your daily routine. This can mean waking up earlier to exercise, taking a break during work to go for a walk, or scheduling a workout before or after work.

Lack of motivation can be addressed by finding an exercise routine that you enjoy and that fits your interests and preferences. Varying your workouts and incorporating new activities can also help to keep things fresh and exciting.

If you are struggling with low energy levels, it's important to assess your diet and sleep habits. Eating a balanced diet and getting enough sleep can help to improve energy levels and make it easier to stick to an exercise routine.

Another common obstacle is injury or illness. It's important to listen to your body and take the necessary time to recover. If you are dealing with an injury, consult with a medical professional to develop a safe and effective exercise plan.

Ultimately, overcoming obstacles requires a combination of perseverance, creativity, and adaptability. By staying focused on your goals and developing strategies to overcome obstacles, you can achieve long-term success in your fitness journey.

V. Key Components of a Sustainable Fitness Routine

- **Recognizing the importance of rest and recovery in preventing burnout**

Rest and recovery are important components of any fitness routine, but they are often overlooked in favor of intense workouts and pushing oneself to the limit. However, without adequate rest and recovery, the body can quickly become fatigued and injury-prone, leading to setbacks in achieving fitness goals.

Rest can take many forms, from taking a day off from exercise to getting enough sleep each night. Recovery, on the other hand, refers to activities that help the body repair and rebuild after a workout, such as stretching, foam rolling, and massage.

Recognizing the importance of rest and recovery can help prevent burnout and injury, allowing individuals to sustain their fitness routine over the long term. It's important to listen to your body and give it the rest and recovery it needs to function at its best.

- **Incorporating mindfulness practices, such as meditation or deep breathing, into your**

routine to   reduce stress and increase focus

Incorporating mindfulness practices, such as meditation or deep breathing, into your routine can help reduce stress and increase focus, which in turn can improve motivation and help you overcome obstacles. Mindfulness practices can also help increase self-awareness and improve overall well-being. By taking a few minutes each day to focus on your breath and quiet your mind, you can become more centered and better equipped to tackle challenges that may arise on your fitness journey. Additionally, practicing mindfulness can help you become more in tune with your body, allowing you to better understand its needs and adjust your workouts or rest days accordingly.

- **Adjusting your approach as needed, and being willing to try new things to keep yourself**

engaged and motivated

Adjusting your approach as needed, and being willing to try new things to keep yourself engaged and motivated is an essential part of staying on track with your fitness goals. Sometimes, even the most dedicated individuals can hit a plateau or lose motivation. In such situations, it may be necessary to switch up your routine or try new activities to reignite your passion for fitness.

Additionally, it's crucial to recognize that setbacks or failures are a normal part of the journey towards better health and fitness. Rather than getting discouraged by setbacks, learn from them and use them as an opportunity to improve and grow. Remember to be kind and patient with yourself, and avoid comparing yourself to others.

Finally, it's essential to prioritize rest and recovery as part of your overall fitness plan. Taking breaks to allow your body to rest and recover can help prevent burnout and injury, and actually lead to better results over time. Incorporating mindfulness practices, such as meditation or deep breathing, can also help reduce stress and increase focus, improving your overall well-being and helping you stay motivated to achieve your goals.

CHAPTER 7

Maintaining Weight Loss and Preventing Relapse

I. Introduction

- Importance of weight loss maintenance
- Challenges of weight loss maintenance

II. Creating a Supportive Environment

- Surrounding yourself with positive influences
- Finding a support system
- Staying accountable

III. Sticking to Healthy Habits

- Consistency in exercise routine
- Making healthy food choices
- Balancing calorie intake and expenditure
- Staying hydrated

IV. Addressing Emotional Eating

- Identifying triggers
- Finding alternative coping mechanisms
- Seeking professional help when needed

V. Coping with Setbacks and Challenges

- Recognizing and learning from mistakes
- Dealing with plateaus
- Overcoming weight loss plateaus
- Dealing with negative self-talk

VI. Keeping the Motivation and Momentum Going

- Setting new goals
- Rewarding yourself for accomplishments
- Celebrating progress

I. Introduction

Maintaining weight loss and preventing relapse can be a challenging task for many individuals who have successfully shed some extra pounds. While losing weight is certainly a significant achievement, the real challenge comes in keeping that weight off over the long term. The key to maintaining weight loss is adopting healthy lifestyle habits that are sustainable and enjoyable. This chapter will discuss various strategies for maintaining weight loss and preventing relapse, including establishing a support system, setting realistic goals, tracking progress, and adjusting your approach as needed. With dedication and commitment, it is possible to maintain weight loss and prevent relapse for a healthier, happier life.

- **Importance of weight loss maintenance**

Maintaining weight loss is an important aspect of long-term health and well-being. Achieving weight loss goals is a significant accomplishment, but it is equally important to keep the weight off in order to avoid health complications and prevent relapse. Unfortunately, many people who successfully lose weight end up regaining it, often due to a lack of sustainable habits and ongoing support. Therefore, developing strategies to maintain weight loss and prevent relapse is crucial for overall health and well-being. In this chapter, we will explore various methods to help you maintain your weight loss and avoid returning to old habits.

- **Challenges of weight loss maintenance**

Maintaining weight loss can be challenging for many individuals. After achieving their weight loss goals, many people find it difficult to sustain the healthy habits that helped them lose weight in the first place. This can lead to weight regain and frustration, which can ultimately result in a return to unhealthy habits and relapse. There are several challenges associated with weight loss maintenance, including the tendency for the body to resist further weight loss, a decrease in motivation and support, and difficulty in sticking to healthy habits in the face of life stressors and temptations. In order to successfully maintain weight loss, it is important to develop strategies for overcoming these challenges and staying committed to healthy lifestyle choices over the long-term.

II. Creating a Supportive Environment

- **Surrounding yourself with positive influences**

Surrounding yourself with positive influences can be a powerful tool in maintaining weight loss. This can include seeking out supportive friends and family members, joining a fitness group or club, or enlisting the help of a professional coach. By surrounding yourself with people who share your goals and encourage your progress, you are more likely to stay motivated and committed to your healthy habits. In addition to social support, it is also important to create an environment that is conducive to maintaining your weight loss. This can include making healthy food choices readily available at home, finding ways to incorporate physical activity into your daily routine, and avoiding environments that may trigger unhealthy habits or behaviors.

By creating a positive and supportive environment, you are setting yourself up for success in maintaining your weight loss and preventing relapse.

- **Finding a support system**

Finding a support system is crucial for maintaining weight loss. This could include family, friends, or a support group. Having people around who are supportive of your goals and can help hold you accountable can make a significant difference in your success. Additionally, having someone to celebrate your successes and encourage you during challenging times can provide the motivation needed to stay on track. Consider joining a support group or working with a personal trainer or coach who can help you stay accountable and provide guidance and motivation.

- **Staying accountable**

Staying accountable is a crucial aspect of maintaining weight loss. This involves continuing to track progress, monitor food intake, and engage in regular physical activity. Accountability can come in many forms, such as partnering with a friend or family member for regular check-ins, joining a weight loss support group, or working with a professional coach. The key is to find a system that works for you and provides the support and motivation needed to stay on track. By holding yourself accountable, you are more likely to stick to healthy habits and prevent relapse.

III. Sticking to Healthy Habits

- **Consistency in exercise routine**

Maintaining a consistent exercise routine is crucial for weight loss maintenance. It's important to continue regular exercise even after reaching your weight loss goals to prevent weight regain. Aim for at least 30 minutes of moderate-intensity exercise most days of the week. Finding an exercise routine that you enjoy and can stick to long-term is key. Mixing up your workouts to prevent boredom and maintain interest can also help you stay consistent. Incorporating strength training can also be beneficial in maintaining weight loss, as it helps build lean muscle mass which can increase your metabolic rate.

- **Making healthy food choices**

Making healthy food choices is a crucial aspect of maintaining weight loss. After achieving weight loss goals, it is important to continue making healthy food choices to prevent weight regain. This involves incorporating a balanced diet that is rich in nutrient-dense foods such as fruits, vegetables, whole grains, lean proteins, and healthy fats while limiting processed foods, sugary drinks, and high-fat foods.

To make healthy food choices, it can be helpful to plan meals in advance, keep healthy snacks on hand, and avoid skipping meals. Additionally, being mindful of portion sizes and using techniques such as mindful eating can also be helpful in maintaining healthy eating habits. It is important to remember that making healthy food choices does not have to be overly restrictive or complicated, and finding a balance that is sustainable for the long-term is key to maintaining weight loss.

- **Balancing calorie intake and expenditure**

Balancing calorie intake and expenditure is an important aspect of weight loss maintenance. To maintain weight loss, it's important to consume the appropriate amount of calories based on your age, gender, activity level, and other factors. Eating too many calories can lead to weight gain, while consuming too few calories can slow down your metabolism and make it harder to maintain weight loss.

It's also important to balance calorie intake with calorie expenditure through physical activity. This means engaging in regular exercise to burn calories and maintain muscle mass. Strength training can also help increase muscle mass and boost metabolism, making it easier to maintain weight loss.

Finding the right balance between calorie intake and expenditure can take time and may require some trial and error. Consulting a healthcare professional or registered dietitian can be helpful in determining the appropriate calorie intake for weight loss maintenance and developing a sustainable exercise plan.

- **Staying hydrated**

Staying hydrated is important for overall health, but it can also play a role in weight loss maintenance. Drinking enough water can help regulate appetite, reduce calorie intake, and increase feelings of fullness. In addition, proper hydration supports exercise performance and recovery. It is recommended that adults drink at least 8 cups (64 ounces) of water per day, but this may vary based on individual needs and activity levels. Other beverages, such as unsweetened tea or infused water, can also contribute to hydration.

IV. Addressing Emotional Eating

- **Identifying triggers**

Identifying triggers is an important step in maintaining weight loss and preventing relapse. Triggers can be anything that causes you to overeat or make unhealthy choices, such as stress, boredom, or social situations. By identifying your triggers, you can develop strategies to avoid or cope with them. For example, if stress is a trigger, you can develop healthy coping mechanisms, such as exercise or meditation, to manage your stress levels. If social situations are a trigger, you can plan ahead by bringing healthy snacks or suggesting a physical activity instead of going out for food and drinks.

- **Finding alternative coping mechanisms**

Finding alternative coping mechanisms is an important aspect of maintaining weight loss and preventing relapse. Many people turn to food as a way to cope with stress, anxiety, or other emotions. It is important to identify these triggers and find alternative coping mechanisms that do not involve food. This can include things like exercise, meditation, journaling, talking to a friend or therapist, or engaging in a favorite hobby. It is also important to develop healthy ways to manage stress and emotions, as this can help prevent relapse and improve overall well-being.

- **Seeking professional help when needed**

Seeking professional help can be an important step in maintaining weight loss and preventing relapse. A healthcare provider, registered dietitian, or certified personal trainer can provide guidance and support to help individuals navigate challenges and make sustainable lifestyle changes. They can also help develop personalized strategies and plans based on individual needs and goals. In addition, seeking support from a therapist or counselor can be beneficial in addressing any underlying emotional or psychological factors that may contribute to overeating or unhealthy habits. It is important to recognize that seeking help is a sign of strength and can lead to greater success in achieving and maintaining weight loss goals.

V. Coping with Setbacks and Challenges

- **Recognizing and learning from mistakes**

Recognizing and learning from mistakes is a process of acknowledging and understanding the errors or misjudgments we have made in the past, and using that knowledge to make better decisions and actions in the future. It involves self-reflection, acceptance of responsibility, and a willingness to grow and improve.

The first step in recognizing and learning from mistakes is acknowledging that they have occurred. This means being honest with ourselves about the choices we have made and the consequences that have resulted from those choices. It may also involve seeking feedback from others who have been affected by our actions.

Once we have recognized our mistakes, the next step is to take responsibility for them. This means not blaming others or making excuses, but instead owning up to our part in the situation and accepting any consequences that may come as a result.

The final step is to learn from our mistakes and use that knowledge to make better decisions in the future. This may involve reflecting on what we could have done differently, seeking out new information or perspectives, or developing new skills or habits to help us avoid similar mistakes in the future.

Recognizing and learning from mistakes is a key aspect of personal and professional growth. By acknowledging our mistakes, taking responsibility for our actions, and using what we have learned to make better decisions, we can become more effective, empathetic, and successful individuals.

- **Dealing with plateaus**

A plateau refers to a period of time in which progress towards a goal or desired outcome seems to stall or slow down, despite consistent effort and hard work. This can be frustrating and demotivating, and it's important to have strategies in place to deal with these types of situations. Here are some tips for dealing with plateaus:

1. Reevaluate your goals and approach: It may be helpful to take a step back and reevaluate your goals and the approach you are taking to achieve them. Are you still working towards the right goals? Do you need to adjust your approach or strategy?
2. Change things up: Sometimes, a change in routine or approach can help break through a plateau. This could involve trying a new workout routine, seeking out new learning resources, or connecting with a mentor or coach.
3. Celebrate small wins: Even if progress towards a larger goal has stalled, it's important to celebrate small wins and successes along the way. This can help you stay motivated and focused on the bigger picture.
4. Take a break: Sometimes, taking a short break or stepping away from a project can help you gain new perspective and energy when you return to it.
5. Stay positive and persistent: It's important to stay positive and keep a growth mindset when dealing with plateaus. Remember that setbacks and obstacles are a normal part of any journey, and that persistence and hard work will ultimately pay off in the long run.

By implementing these strategies, you can navigate plateaus and continue to make progress towards your goals.

- **Overcoming weight loss plateaus**

Weight loss plateaus can be frustrating, but they are a common part of the weight loss journey. The body has a natural tendency to adapt to changes, including changes in diet and exercise, which can result in a slowdown in weight loss progress. However, there are several strategies that can be effective in overcoming weight loss plateaus.

1. Increase physical activity: If you have been following the same exercise routine for a while, your body may have adapted to it, resulting in a plateau. You can break through the plateau by increasing the intensity or duration of your workouts. Consider adding weight training, high-intensity interval training (HIIT), or increasing the duration of your cardio workouts.
2. Adjust your diet: Sometimes, small adjustments to your diet can help break a weight loss plateau. For example, you can try reducing your caloric intake by a small amount or increasing your protein intake to help preserve muscle mass.
3. Keep track of your food intake: Keeping a food diary or using a food tracking app can help you become more aware of what you are eating and how much you are eating. This can help you identify areas where you can make changes and keep yourself accountable.
4. Get enough sleep: Sleep is essential for weight loss and overall health. Lack of sleep can lead to hormonal imbalances that can make weight loss more difficult. Aim for seven to eight hours of sleep each night.
5. Manage stress: Stress can lead to overeating and hinder weight loss progress. Find healthy ways to manage stress, such as yoga, meditation, or deep breathing exercises.

6. Consider professional help: If you have been struggling with a weight loss plateau for an extended period, consider seeking the help of a healthcare professional, such as a registered dietitian or a personal trainer. They can provide personalized recommendations and support to help you overcome the plateau.

Remember, weight loss is a journey, and there may be setbacks and plateaus along the way. Stay focused on your goals, be patient, and keep making healthy choices, and you will eventually break through the plateau and continue making progress towards your goals.

- **Dealing with negative self-talk**

Negative self-talk is the inner dialogue that we have with ourselves, which can be critical and damaging to our self-esteem and mental health. It is often characterized by thoughts that are self-defeating, self-critical, and irrational. Dealing with negative self-talk requires self-awareness, self-compassion, and a willingness to challenge and change negative thought patterns. Here are some strategies that can help:

1. Identify negative self-talk: The first step in dealing with negative self-talk is to become aware of when it is happening. Take note of the negative thoughts that come to mind, and try to recognize any patterns or triggers.
2. Challenge negative self-talk: Once you have identified negative self-talk, challenge it by questioning its validity. Ask yourself if there is any evidence to support the negative thought, and if not, try to replace it with a more positive and realistic thought.
3. Practice self-compassion: It is essential to treat yourself with kindness and compassion. Avoid harsh self-criticism and instead, focus on self-acceptance and self-love. Try to talk to yourself as you would a close friend, with encouragement and empathy.
4. Reframe negative thoughts: Reframe negative thoughts by focusing on the positive aspects of a situation. Instead of dwelling on what went wrong, try to focus on what you learned or what you can do differently in the future.
5. Surround yourself with positivity: Surround yourself with positive people, and engage in activities that bring you joy and fulfillment. This can help counteract negative self-talk and boost your self-esteem.
6. Seek professional help: If negative self-talk is impacting your daily life and mental health, consider seeking the help of a mental health professional, such as a therapist. They can provide personalized support and strategies to help you overcome negative self-talk and improve your mental well-being.

Remember that overcoming negative self-talk takes time and effort, but with practice and persistence, you can change your thought patterns and improve your self-esteem and mental health.

VI. Keeping the Motivation and Momentum Going

- **Setting new goals**

Setting new goals in weight loss can help you stay motivated and on track with your weight loss journey. Here are some steps to help you set new goals:

1. Assess your progress: Before setting new goals, take the time to assess your progress so far. Reflect on your successes, challenges, and areas for improvement. This will help you identify what you need to focus on moving forward.
2. Define specific, measurable goals: To set new goals, it's important to define specific and measurable objectives. For example, instead of saying you want to lose weight, set a specific goal, such as losing 5 pounds in the next month. This makes it easier to track your progress and stay motivated.
3. Make your goals challenging but achievable: Your goals should be challenging enough to push you out of your comfort zone but also achievable. Set goals that are realistic based on your current health and fitness level, and make sure to break them down into smaller milestones that are easier to achieve.
4. Consider a variety of goals: In addition to weight loss goals, consider setting goals related to other areas of health and wellness, such as increasing your physical activity, eating more fruits and vegetables, reducing stress, and improving sleep quality.
5. Create an action plan: Once you have defined your goals, create an action plan that outlines the steps you need to take to achieve them. This can include specific diet and exercise changes, tracking your progress, and seeking support from friends, family, or a healthcare professional.
6. Celebrate your successes: Finally, remember to celebrate your successes along the way. Recognize and reward yourself for achieving milestones and staying on track with your goals. This can help you stay motivated and committed to your weight loss journey.

Setting new goals in weight loss can help you stay focused, motivated, and committed to achieving your desired outcomes. By following these steps, you can create achievable goals that will help you reach your weight loss and wellness goals.

- **Rewarding yourself for accomplishments**

Rewarding yourself for accomplishments in weight loss is an important way to stay motivated and encouraged as you work towards your goals. Here are some tips for rewarding yourself for your weight loss accomplishments:

1. Choose rewards that align with your goals: When choosing rewards, select those that support your weight loss goals. For example, if your goal is to exercise more, consider rewarding yourself with a new workout outfit or a fitness tracker.

2. Make rewards meaningful to you: Choose rewards that are meaningful and enjoyable for you. For instance, if you love to read, reward yourself with a new book or a magazine subscription.
3. Set specific milestones: Set specific milestones for your weight loss journey, such as losing 5 pounds or completing a specific fitness challenge. This will help you stay focused and motivated.
4. Celebrate non-scale victories: Remember that weight loss is not just about the number on the scale. Celebrate non-scale victories such as increased energy, improved mood, and better sleep.
5. Don't use food as a reward: Avoid using food as a reward, as this can lead to unhealthy eating habits. Instead, choose rewards that support your health and wellness goals.
6. Consider social rewards: Social rewards can be especially motivating. Plan a fun outing with friends or family to celebrate your accomplishments.
7. Make rewards attainable: Ensure that the rewards you choose are attainable and within your budget. This will help you stay motivated without causing financial stress.

Remember, rewarding yourself for your accomplishments in weight loss is a great way to stay motivated and encouraged on your journey. By choosing rewards that align with your goals, are meaningful to you, and celebrate both scale and non-scale victories, you can stay committed to achieving your goals and creating a healthier lifestyle.

- **Celebrating progress**

Celebrating progress in weight loss is an essential part of maintaining motivation and staying committed to your goals. Here are some ways to celebrate your progress in weight loss:

1. Track your progress: Keep track of your progress using a journal or an app that records your weight, measurements, and other relevant data. Tracking your progress can help you see how far you have come and provide motivation to keep going.
2. Celebrate small victories: Celebrate small victories along the way, such as losing a pound, fitting into a smaller size, or making it through a week without giving in to temptation. Take time to acknowledge and celebrate these achievements to help stay motivated and encouraged.
3. Reward yourself: Set rewards for yourself as you reach specific milestones, such as a new workout outfit, a massage, or a weekend getaway. Choose rewards that are meaningful to you and align with your values and interests.
4. Share your progress: Share your progress with friends and family who are supportive and encouraging. Celebrate your achievements with them, and allow them to cheer you on as you continue to work towards your goals.
5. Focus on non-scale victories: Remember that progress in weight loss is not just about the number on the scale. Celebrate non-scale victories such as increased energy, improved mood, better sleep, and improved overall health.

6. Reflect on your journey: Take time to reflect on your weight loss journey and acknowledge the hard work you have put in. Think about the challenges you have overcome, the healthy habits you have developed, and the positive changes you have made.

Remember that weight loss is a journey, and progress is not always linear. Celebrating your progress along the way can help you stay motivated, focused, and committed to achieving your goals. By celebrating small victories, rewarding yourself, sharing your progress, focusing on non-scale victories, and reflecting on your journey, you can stay motivated and encouraged as you work towards a healthier lifestyle.

References

The Ultimate Guide to Successful Weight Loss. (2023, June 18). Retrieved from https://openai.com/blog/chatgpt

Douglas, W. (2023, February 21). *LOSING WEIGHT, THE HEALTHY WAY: Practical Tips and Strategies for Sustainable Weight Loss*. Barnesandnoble. https://www.barnesandnoble.com/w/losing-weight-the-healthy-way-wesley-douglas/1143131154

Martinez, D. (2023, April 23). *Man Down: The Weight Loss Bible for Men*. Goodreads. https://www.goodreads.com/book/show/139397542-man-down

Ferreira, J. (2022, December 8). *Exploring the Different Types of Career Coaching and How to Become a Career Coach*. Careersuccesspartner. https://www.careersuccesspartner.com/career/best-career-coaching/

Ptak, D. (2019, March 1). *Traditional Fundraising Programs Pros/Cons*. Linkedin. https://www.linkedin.com/pulse/traditional-fundraising-programs-proscons-dan-ptak

Paparan, J. C. (2023, April 27). *Paparan Jitendra Chouksey*. Linkedin. https://my.linkedin.com/posts/jitendrachouksey_way-too-many-supplements-claiming-to-fix-activity-7057264407474507776-cHlU

Anthony, P. (2023, February 27). *A Weight Loss Coach Can Help You Reframe Your Mindset for better results*. Paulanthony. https://paulanthony.ca/blog/A+Weight+Loss+Coach+Can+Help+You+Reframe+Your+Mindset+For+Better+Results/362#:~:text=The%20Importance%20of%20Mindset%20in%20Weight%20Loss

Dhakad, A. (n.d.). *Will skipping meals reduce weight?* Quora. https://www.quora.com/Will-skipping-meals-reduce-weight

How Long till You See Weight Loss. (2023, April 19). Retrieved from https://tellmechina.com/health/2023/04/19/en-how-long-till-you-see-weight-loss/

The Number 1 Exercise for Losing Unwanted Body Fat. (2023, March 24). Retrieved from https://www.boxrox.com/the-number-1-exercise-for-losing-unwanted-body-fat/#:~:text=What%20is%20a%20Calorie%20Deficit,through%20exercise%20and%20physical%20activity

Braverman, J. (2018, November 28). *Can You Eat Less & Gain Weight?* Weekand. https://www.weekand.com/healthy-living/article/can-eat-less-gain-weight-18005481.php

Smith, L. (2023, March 7). *Is it possible to lose weight with exercise alone and not really focusing on diet? How much would a 90kg person have to exercise a day to lose 20kgs?* Quora. https://www.quora.com/Is-it-possible-to-lose-weight-with-exercise-alone-and-not-really-focusing-on-diet-How-much-would-a-90kg-person-have-to-exercise-a-day-to-lose-20kgs/log

Why do people say that "calories don't matter when losing weight"?. (2023, March 13). Retrieved from https://www.quora.com/Why-do-people-say-that-calories-don-t-matter-when-losing-weight

At what age do you start gaining fat?. (n.d.). Retrieved from https://www.coalitionbrewing.com/at-what-age-do-you-start-gaining-fat/

Terry, S. (n.d.). *Https://ketoacvgummies.Com/tot....Al-health-acv-keto-g*. Topicfx. https://topicfx.com/post/19129

Messina, M. (n.d.). *Achieving Your Goals*. Drmessina. https://www.drmessina.com/blog/achieving-your-goals

McGuire, S. (2013, September 5). Ncbi.nlm.nih. https://www.ncbi.nlm.nih.gov/pmc/articles/PMC3771156/

Report-0.22780300 1684194449

Sang, M. (2023, March 11). *The art of meal prepping: Time-saving tips for busy families*. Tastetutorial. https://tastetutorial.com/the-art-of-meal-prepping-time-saving-tips-for-busy-families/

Caudill, A. (2014, September 5). *Scientists at University of Oregon Link Running to Sensory Processing*. Info.Biotech-Calendar. https://info.biotech-calendar.com/Biotechnology-Calendar-Company-Events-and-News/bid/112976/Scientists-at-University-of-Oregon-Link-Running-to-Sensory-Processing

Which is more important diet or exercise?. (2023, April 16). Retrieved from https://worldwisewebstories.com/which-is-more-important-diet-or-exercise/#:~:text=of%20well%2Dbeing.-,Regular%20physical%20exercise%20provides%20numerous%20benefits%20for%20overall%20health%20and,energy%20levels%2C%20improved%20cognitive%20function%2C

The Importance of Regular Exercise for a Healthy Life. (2023, May 4). Retrieved from https://www.freelancer.com/projects/typing/typing-typing-grammar-mistake-content

Science of Weight Loss. (n.d.). Retrieved from https://www.elevatingevolution.com/about-5

7 benefits of regular physical activity. (2021, October 8). Retrieved from https://www.mayoclinic.org/healthy-lifestyle/fitness/in-depth/exercise/art-20048389

Cotton, A. (2022, January 3). *All About Metabolism Part 1: Five Things You Must Know*. Alexandriastylebook. https://alexandriastylebook.com/alexandria-stylebook/all-about-metabolism-part1-five-things-you-must-know-alexandriawellness-january-2022

How to lose weight. (2023, April 28). Retrieved from https://amazoneasystore.com/how-to-loose-weight/

Serranti, M. (n.d.). *57 personal trainer vicino a te*. Starofservice. https://www.starofservice.it/dir/umbria/terni/terni/personal-training

Importance of exercise for seniors. (2023, February 19). Retrieved from https://www.seniorfitlife.com/2023/02/what-is-best-exercise-for-70-year-old.html

[A group in a Facebook page that share loss weight ideas]. (n.d.). Facebook. https://www.facebook.com/groups/433037803750213/permalink/1168858820168104

Ptak, D. (2019, March 1). *Traditional Fundraising Programs Pros/Cons*. Linkedin. https://www.linkedin.com/pulse/traditional-fundraising-programs-proscons-dan-ptak

Chouksey, J. (2023, April 27). *Paparan Jitendra Chouksey*. My.Linkedin. https://my.linkedin.com/posts/jitendrachouksey_way-too-many-supplements-claiming-to-fix-activity-7057264407474507776-cHlU

[A group in Quora website that share loss weight ideas]. (n.d.). Quora. https://www.quora.com/Will-skipping-meals-reduce-weight

The Number 1 Exercise for Losing Unwanted Body Fat. (2023, March 24). Retrieved from https://www.boxrox.com/the-number-1-exercise-for-losing-unwanted-body-fat/#:~:text=What%20is%20a%20Calorie%20Deficit,through%20exercise%20and%20physical%20activity

Smith, L. (2022, March 7). *Is it possible to lose weight with exercise alone and not really focusing on diet? How much would a 90kg person have to exercise a day to lose 20kgs?* Quora. https://www.quora.com/Is-it-possible-to-lose-weight-with-exercise-alone-and-not-really-focusing-on-diet-How-much-would-a-90kg-person-have-to-exercise-a-day-to-lose-20kgs

STAYING MOTIVATED WHEN EXERCISING. (2023, March 10). Retrieved from https://www.emeryphysicaltherapy.com/blog/STAYING-MOTIVATED-WHEN-EXERCISING~14312.html

Helping a Family Member Who Has PTSD. (2023, April 20). Retrieved from https://veteransnavigator.org/article/13032/helping-family-member-who-has-ptsd

How to Lose Weight Fast: 7 Proven Strategies for Quick Results. (2023, May 3). Retrieved from https://www.corenutri.com/2023/05/03/how-to-lose-weight-fast-7-proven-strategies-for-quick-results.html#:~:text=It's%20also%20important%20to%20remember,into%20account%20when%20setting%20goals.

Mulik, P. (n.d.). *Should exercise be the only component of a weight loss plan?* Quora. https://www.quora.com/Should-exercise-be-the-only-component-of-a-weight-loss-plan

Narang, S. (n.d.). *Take individual responsibility to attain optimal health*. Linkedin. https://ma.linkedin.com/posts/simranarang19651988_take-individual-responsibility-to-attain-activity-7050695436487012352-ale3

The benefits of regular exercise for weight management & overall health. (n.d.). Retrieved from https://prblonde.com/the-benefits-of-healthy-a-lifestyle-and-weight

Echoda, D. (2023, April 16). *Frequent Hunger as a UI Student: Causes and Remedies*. Indypressui. https://indypressui.org/2023/04/16/frequent-hunger-as-a-ui-student-causes-and-remedies/

Making Mental Health a Priority: Science-Backed Strategies for Self-Care. 8.Health. (2022, June 22). Retrieved from https://8.health/blogs/news/making-mental-wellness-a-priority

Weight Gain Meal Plan. (n.d.). Retrieved from https://dubaipt.com/meal-plans/weight-gain-diet/

Joana, F. (2022, December 8). *Exploring the Different Types of Career Coaching and How to Become a Career Coach*. Careersuccesspartner. https://www.careersuccesspartner.com/career/best-career-coaching/

How to maintain a healthy lifestyle. (2023, January 4). Retrieved from https://topentise.com/how-to-maintain-a-healthy-lifestyle

Akeem, C. (2023, February 19). *Compassionate Approaches to Weight Loss: Small Changes for Big Impact*. Health3wellness. https://health3wellness.com/mindset/compassionate-approaches-to-weight-loss-small-changes-for-big-impact/

Jumani, M. (n.d.). *Ana Navarro's Workout Routine: How She Stays Fit The Importance of Fitness in Ana Navarro's Life*. Vocal.Media. https://vocal.media/longevity/ana-navarro-s-workout-routine-how-she-stays-fit

Smith, M. (n.d.). *Male Successfully Loses Weight: A Weight Journey on Reddit*. Myprogresspics. https://myprogresspics.com/progress-pics/13854/male-successfully-loses-weight-a-weight-journey-on-reddit

THE SCIENCE BEHIND EPOC: HOW THE AFTERBURN EFFECT BOOSTS YOUR METABOLISM. (2022, December 27). Retrieved from https://plutoniqfitness.com/the-science-behind-epoc-boosts-your-metabolism/

Tergar'S Effective Approach To Stress Reduction Techniques. (2023, February 26). Retrieved from https://healthupdatesfresh.com/tergar-learning-tergars-effective-approach-to-stress-reduction-techniques/

Raise Capital without sacrificing Control of Your Startup. (2023, March 9). Retrieved from https://fastercapital.com/content/Raise-Capital-without-sacrificing-Control-of-Your-Startup.html

JAVED, I. (n.d.). *The Extreme Weight Cutting and Hydration Secrets of UFC Fighters*. Vocal.Media. https://vocal.media/education/the-extreme-weight-cutting-and-hydration-secrets-of-ufc-fighters-aibzaa0702

SIDE STITCH WHEN RUNNING: CAUSES, PREVENTION, AND TREATMENT. (2023, May 6). Retrieved from https://sportcoaching.co.nz/side-stitch-when-running/

Sheree-Ann, M. (2023, April 14). *7 Simple and Sustainable Habits for Getting- and Staying-Motivated!* Linkedin. https://www.linkedin.com/pulse/7-simple-sustainable-habits-getting-michelle-bpharm-fmchc

Christopher, L. (2023, May 9). *How to Stay Motivated as a Leader*. Changemylifecoaching.ca. https://changemylifecoaching.ca/2023/05/09/stay-motivated-as-a-leader/#:~:text=By%20setting%20clear%20goals%2C%20celebrating,stay%20motivated%20and%20become%20a

The Wellness whisperer. (n.d.). Retrieved from https://wellnesswhisperer.blogspot.com/2023/03/what-is-balanced-diet.html

Aishwarya, A. (n.d.). *Is Orange Good For Weight Loss? Get The Answer You've Been Waiting For.* Fitelo. https://fitelo.co/is-orange-good-for-weight-loss/

Top 10 Health Benefits of Mushrooms, the Ultimate Superfood. (2022, August 16). Retrieved from https://scitechdaily.com/top-10-health-benefits-of-mushrooms-the-ultimate-superfood/

Bedosky, L. (2020, March 10). *5 Best Workouts For Fat Loss, Ranked*. Blog.Myfitnesspal. https://blog.myfitnesspal.com/5-best-exercises-for-fat-loss-ranked/

The benefits of healthy a lifestyle and wheight. (n.d.). Retrieved from https://prblonde.com/the-benefits-of-healthy-a-lifestyle-and-weight

Braveman, J. (n.d.). *Can You Lose Lower Back Fat and Love Handles in Two Weeks?* Livestrong. https://www.livestrong.com/article/516561-how-to-lose-lower-back-fat-and-love-handles-in-two-weeks/

Look for the author

Do we have to workout in order for our body to burn calories?. (2023, January 14). Retrieved from https://www.quora.com/Do-we-have-to-workout-in-order-for-our-body-to-burn-calories

Cotton, A. (2022, January 3). *All About Metabolism Part 1: Five Things You Must Know*. Alexandriastylebook. https://alexandriastylebook.com/alexandria-stylebook/all-about-metabolism-part1-five-things-you-must-know-alexandriawellness-january-2022*STRENGTH TRAINING*. (n.d.). Retrieved from https://natefit.ca/fitness-lifestyle-blog/strength-training

10 Best Exercises And Their Benefits. (2023, April 24). Retrieved from https://oceanofimages.com/exercise/

Boost Your Brainpower: The Benefits of Exercise for Improved Cognitive Function and Memory. (n.d.). Retrieved from https://www.americansportandfitness.com/blogs/fitness-blog/boost-your-brainpower-the-benefits-of-exercise-for-improved-cognitive-function-and-memory

The Easy Way to Memorizing Scripture. (2023, April 21). Retrieved from https://arabahjoy.com/the-easy-way-to-memorizing-scripture/

A Comprehensive Guide About Exercise. Kips-Media. (2023, February 18). Retrieved from https://www.kips-media.com/a-comprehensive-guide-about-exercise/

What are tips for weight loss?. (2023, April 2). Retrieved from https://www.quora.com/profile/Ajay-4192

Goal setting. (n.d.). Retrieved from https://www.studocu.com/en-us/document/henry-ford-college/personal-finance/chapter-1-goal-setting/49849451

Aglawe, V. (n.d.). *Goal Setting - Gold or Gimmick?* Linkedin. https://al.linkedin.com/posts/vikrantaglawe_goalsetting-objectives-okrs-activity-7032243414645551104-1WQ6

20 Simple Techniques to Prioritizing and Clarifying Your Goals for Success. (2023, March 23). Retrieved from https://effizone.com/20-simple-techniques-to-prioritizing-and-clarifying-your-goals-for-success/

The importance of tracking your progress when losing weight. (2023, February 26). Retrieved from https://www.fitlivingtips.co.in/2023/02/the-importance-of-tracking-your.html

How to Overcome Obstacles and Achieve Your Goals. (2023, February 25). Retrieved from https://dripsuccess.com/f/how-to-overcome-obstacles-and-achieve-your-goals

How to Lose Weight at Home: Tips and Tricks for Effective Weight Loss. (2023, May 4). Retrieved from https://gsmteng.com/how-to-lose-weight-at-home/

Top 10 Fat Loss Tips. (2023, May 13). Retrieved from https://sonowalstory.blogspot.com/2023/05/Top%2010%20Fat%20Loss%20Tips.html

Smith, M. (n.d.). *Male Successfully Loses Weight: A Weight Journey on Reddit.* Myprogresspics. https://myprogresspics.com/progress-pics/13854/male-successfully-loses-weight-a-weight-journey-on-reddit

Johnson, J. (2023, January 22). *What long-term strategies can help me maintain a healthy weight?* Quora. https://www.quora.com/What-long-term-strategies-can-help-me-maintain-a-healthy-weight

How a Clean Home Can Improve Your Overall Well-being. (n.d.). Retrieved from https://walkingfruitfully.com/how-a-clean-home-can-improve-your-overall-well-being/

Jasso, R. (2023, May 1). *Breaking the Cycle: Strategies for Transforming Dysfunctional Family Relationships.* Talksovercoffee. https://www.talksovercoffee.com/blog/breaking-the-cycle-strategies-for-transforming-dysfunctional-family-relationships

Benefit Of Exercise In Old Age. (2023, March 27). Retrieved from https://painrehab.org/f/benefit-of-exercise-in-old-age

20 Tips For Staying Healthy In Your 20s. (2023, March 17). Retrieved from https://twentiesandthriving.com/20-tips-for-staying-healthy-in-your-20s/

[A blog website that lists weight loss information]. (n.d.). fitnesspoint711.blogspot. https://fitnesspoint711.blogspot.com/2023/05/Regular-Exercise-For-Fitness%20.html

Sam, W. (2023, February 13). *The Benefits of Outdoor Exercise and How to Incorporate it into Your Workout Routine.* Healthyleanhabits. https://healthyleanhabits.com/benefits-of-outdoor-exercise-incorporating-into-workout-routine

10 Nutritious Meals for Women's Weight Loss Journey. (2023, May 6). Retrieved from https://vocal.media/lifehack/10-nutritious-meals-for-women-s-weight-loss-journey

Echoda , D. (2023, April 16). *Frequent Hunger as a UI Student: Causes and Remedies*. Indypressui. https://indypressui.org/2023/04/16/frequent-hunger-as-a-ui-student-causes-and-remedies/

Maximizing Brain Performance: Tips and Strategies. (n.d.). Retrieved from https://www.zentein.ca/post/maximizing-brain-performance-tips-and-strategies

Stress management. (2020, October 14). Retrieved from https://www.theprivatesea.com.au/post/stress-management

Gope, M. (2023, March 12). *Stress managment and coping strategies*. Slideshare. https://www.slideshare.net/MonojitGope/stress-managementpptx-256413574

Unlocking the Power of Sleep: How Prioritizing Rest Enhances Brain Function and Emotional Wellbeing. (2023, April 8). Retrieved from https://sleeprecharged.com/blogs/news/unlocking-the-power-of-sleep-how-prioritizing-rest-enhances-brain-function-and-emotional-wellbeing

Malik, Y. (2023, May 1). *The Importance of Sleep for Your Health: Benefits and Consequences of Good and Poor Sleep*. Learnwithyousra. https://learnwithyousra.blogspot.com/2023/05/the-importance-of-sleep-for-your-health_1.html

GETTING QUALITY SLEEP – 9 TIPS & TRICKS. (2023, April 12). Retrieved from https://lovenotestola.com/getting-quality-sleep-9-tips-tricks/?utm_source=rss

Overcoming Fitness Plateaus: The Power of Rest and Nutrition. (n.d.). Retrieved from https://renewgym.co.uk/uncategorized/overcoming-fitness-plateaus-the-power-of-rest-and-nutrition/

What Is a Goal Tree, and Should You Start Using One to Grow Performance? Employee-Performance. (n.d.). Retrieved from https://employee-performance.com/blog/what-is-a-goal-tree/#:~:text=By%20breaking%20down%20larger%20goals,clear%20framework%20for%20decision%2Dmaking.

Denby, S. (n.d.). Facebook. https://www.facebook.com/groups/433037803750213/permalink/1168858820168104

7 Simple Ways to Boost Your Happiness and Well-Being. (n.d.). Retrieved from https://www.inspiredcomforts.com/blogs/news/7-simple-ways-to-boost-your-happiness-and-well-being

Schaefer, G. (2023, March 20). *How To Set And Maintain Goals*. Soulful-Recovery. https://www.soulful-recovery.com/how-to-set-and-maintain-goals/

Maintaining a Healthy Lifestyle. (2022, August 17). Retrieved from https://sportcbds.com/why-is-my-bench-press-so-inconsistent-everything-you-need-to-know/

Patterns of Behavior: What You Should Know About Them. (n.d.). Retrieved from
https://therapymantra.co/self-care/behavior-patterns/

Shockey, D. (2023, April 28). *Depression Is A Common And Serious Medical Illness, But Treatable*.
Tampafp. https://www.tampafp.com/depression-is-a-common-and-serious-medical-illness-but-treatable/

Your new year's guide to quitting smoking in 2023. (n.d.). Retrieved from
https://www.byegwaai.co.za/blog/new-years-guide-to-quitting-smoking-2023

How can I lose 7 pounds in 3 weeks?. (n.d.). Retrieved from https://www.quora.com/How-can-I-lose-7-pounds-in-3-weeks look for author

Tips to improve concentration. (2020, October 1). Retrieved from
https://www.health.harvard.edu/mind-and-mood/tips-to-improve-concentration

Block, A. (n.d.). [linkedin page describing how to achieve those goals]. Linkedin.
https://tz.linkedin.com/posts/andrewjamesblock_businesstips-revfuel-activity-7014593190502547456-D1I-

How to Stay Motivated During Your Weight Loss Journey?. (2023, May 16). Retrieved from
https://womenfitnessmag.com/how-to-stay-motivated-during-your-weight-loss-journey/

How do you reward yourself for completing your tasks and staying productive?. (2023, April 28).
Retrieved from https://www.linkedin.com/advice/3/how-do-you-reward-yourself-completing

How to Build Endurance for Long-Distance Running. (n.d.). Retrieved from
https://www.fitnessframework.co.uk/post/how-to-build-endurance-for-long-distance-running

www.ingramcontent.com/pod-product-compliance
Lightning Source LLC
Chambersburg PA
CBHW080724260726
48660CB00010B/3689